Endless Energy

Free downloads of facilitated exercises from the book are available at
www.EndlessEnergyBook.com.

If you wish to understand the universe
Think of energy, frequency, and vibration.

~ Nikola Tesla

Endless Energy

The Essential Guide to Energy Health

Debra Greene, Ph.D.

MetaComm Media, Maui

METACOMM MEDIA

Published in the United States of America
by MetaComm Media.
1215 S. Kihei Rd. Ste. 0-907
Maui, HI 96753
info@MetaComm.us
www.MetaComm.us

MetaComm Media, 2009 (revised)

ISBN-13: 978-0-615-26933-7
ISBN-10: 0-615-26933-8
LCCN: 2009922855

Printed in the United States of America

Cover photo by Bob Pedersen. Graphic art by Bob Pedersen.

Neither the author nor the publisher is engaged in providing professional advice
or services to the individual reader. The ideas, procedures, and suggestions
contained in this book are not intended to substitute for consulting with a quali-
fied health care provider. Neither the author not the publisher shall be liable or
responsible for any loss or damage allegedly arising from any information or
suggestion contained in this book.

The author has made every effort to provide accurate contact information and
addresses at the time of publication. However, neither the author nor the publisher assumes any responsibility for errors or changes that occur after publication, nor are they responsible for third-party websites or their content.

To my students for being such good teachers.

To my clients for being such good healers.

To my teachers for being such good souls.

Author's Note

I have tried to present a smorgasbord of ideas, with something for everyone. There will be offerings that you savor and others you choose to pass up. Much has gone into the preparation and presentation. I invite you to partake as you choose. Please enjoy the feast.

I gratefully acknowledge
My parents because they don't know,
My friends because they do.

Many over the years have inspired this book. I am deeply indebted to Grethe Fremming and Rolf Havsboel for introducing me to the Ageless Wisdom. My students and clients were the first to ask for a book. Their insightful questions and commitment to conscious growth informed much of its content. My parents created a need for a book so they could understand what I do. I thank them for being interested, especially my step-mom Merle. Friends were kind enough to read drafts of chapters and offer feedback. Sharon Abbondanza and Tricia Morris were supportive in dialoguing with me and understanding when I dropped out of their lives for long periods. I gratefully acknowledge Web guru extraordinaire Jay Ligda (aka lightning god) for careful reading of every line and thoughtful comments on each chapter. I so appreciate Jaime Williams who appeared like an angel from the heavens and swooped down to assist with the book's publicity and promotion. Thanks to editor Alison Gardner for her keen eye, fresh perspective, and enthusiasm for the book, and to Margaret Astrid Phanes for her meditative presence and fingertip finesse with layout and design. Most of all, thank you, dear reader, for your willingness to learn and openness to new ways of being.

Contents

List of Exercises

Chapter One

Understanding Energy

Would you like to have more energy? More zest for life? Put that spring back in your step? The truth is lack of vitality affects everyone at times. You know the feeling. The alarm goes off and you struggle to wake up. Sometimes it seems like you could sleep forever. Life hands you a challenge and you feel too drained to deal with it. Dread seeps in. It's hard to get excited about anything. You try eating better and getting more rest but you still can't seem to bounce back. Where did your energy go?

You get home from work feeling exhausted after a long, intense week and can't wait to take a shower and relax for the evening. The thought of going to bed early sounds very appealing. But then the phone rings. It's a friend you're fond of and haven't seen in awhile. She's in the area for a meeting that ended earlier than expected and she wants to get together. Suddenly you perk up and have more energy than you've had all week. You stay up late talking and enjoying every moment. Where did that energy come from?

We've been told that energy comes from food. If you eat a good, healthy diet you will have more energy. But if energy comes from food then we should be able to eat more and have more energy. Unfortunately, it doesn't work that way. Eating more eventually brings on obesity so we end up overweight and fatigued.

We've also been told that energy comes from adequate exercise and good sleep. But the same logical extension applies. If energy comes from exercise, by exercising constantly we should gain more energy. But we don't. Eventually we lose energy and get exhausted. If energy comes from sleep, by sleeping all the time we should have more energy. But we don't.

We are told it's a question of balancing a healthy diet with adequate exercise and good sleep. If these three factors are in harmony, the body will manufacture energy. But you can sleep, exercise and eat well, yet still feel depleted. Where does the energy go? At times, it's also possible to be deprived of sleep, food, or exercise, yet still feel great. Where does that energy come from?

We are told that energy derives from within our body's cells. A biochemical reaction takes place between the cell's mitochondria and a large molecule called ATP (adenosine triphosphate). ATP is considered the energy source of all living things. It is commonly referred to as the *energy currency* of the cell and is said to be responsible for powering all the activity of your entire system. ATP energy can be converted into electrical energy, into other chemical bonds, or into the power used for movement by the contraction of your muscle cells. This formula is well understood and heavily documented in medical textbooks. If you study any aspect of human health, from a basic high school biology class to becoming a full fledged medical doctor, you will find the same explanation for where energy comes from: a biochemical reaction involving ATP and the cell's mitochondria.

There's just one problem: it doesn't quite work that way. It turns out the ATP explanation is only half true. A new scientific understanding of human energy has emerged in the last few decades that overturned the long established wisdom about how your body works. Compelling research over a span of 15 years by biophysicists shows the energy necessary to power the human body must include some other source.

The Unaccounted For Energy

When Nobel Prize winning biophysicist A.V. Hill looked deeply into the workings of ATP he discovered something missing.[1]

He found that the mitochondria/ATP explanation could not account for all of the energy necessary to power the human body. Although over 60% of the energy needed to function was due to that biochemical interaction, the rest was a mystery. That means almost 40% of the energy was unexplained and could not be attributed to any biological functioning whatsoever. Dr. Hill referred to this as the *unaccounted for* energy and called upon fellow scientists to address the issue.

Support for this invisible energy source has grown to the extent that in 1994 the National Institutes of Health (NIH) formally recognized the existence of a biofield, a *non-physical* energy that surrounds and permeates the human body.[2] This energy is not electromagnetic, infrared, or radio wave. It is something other. Researchers from a variety of fields keep encountering it and so it goes by many names. Sometimes called *subtle energy, etheric energy, zero point energy, epigenetic phenomena,* or *matrix energy,* the consensus is this energy is responsible for a great deal of our functioning.[3] Much has been written about energy from these various perspectives. My goal is not to dispute or support their claims but to take them at face value and describe what this means for you and your energy health.

When energy is brought into the picture many mysteries of the human body find their answers. Although subtle energy greatly impacts health, most of us don't know about it. Somehow this key component has not found its way into mainstream medicine. Because conventional medicine is based solely in the physical sciences, it doesn't allow for anything other than what can be physically observed and measured. To understand the "unaccounted for" energy, we have to go outside the comfort zone of the familiar.

There is a story about a man who lost his keys. It was dark outside and he was frantically searching under a streetlight. A passerby happened upon him and asked, "What are you looking for?" The man replied that he had lost his keys. The passerby then asked, "Where is the last place you saw them?" to which the man replied, "Over there in the park." This prompted the passerby to ask,

"So why aren't you looking over there?" The man replied, "Because the light is better here."

So it is with conventional medical approaches. The keys to unlocking health problems are sought in the physical body because that is familiar and comfortable. When the answers are not to be found, the search continues in the same place and we are told there is simply no explanation. Of course, the answers will never be found if they are sought in the wrong place. The search must be expanded.

Looking at the unresolved issues that plague modern medicine, we can see the need for change. Of all countries in the world, the US ranks tops in health care spending, yet life expectancy is a dismally low forty-first.[4] Health care expenses in 2006 accounted for over 15% of the US gross domestic product. Despite increased costs and advances in health care, more people are suffering from a variety of ailments that range from cancer, heart disease, stroke, autoimmune dysfunctions, and obesity to various forms of mental illness. Children are being medicated at increasingly younger ages for anxiety and attention disorders and the number of Americans with Alzheimer's has doubled since 1980, affecting almost five million adults.[5]

Conflicting health advice has reached epidemic proportions. For every study that advocates a particular healthcare approach, there seems to be another cautioning against it. Mixed messages abound about everything from diet and sun exposure to medical treatments and their side effects. Frustrated and confused, people are responding by taking health matters into their own hands and doing so without medical guidance. A full 62% of participants in a National Institutes for Health survey use alternative approaches to improve their health and the majority do not consult a medical practitioner.[6] Clearly, something is missing when it comes to mainstream health care options, and that "something" can be summed up in one word: energy.

The Vital Force

In spring of 2006 a class of 29 students went on a field trip to Fort Lauderdale Park for their forensics class. To help enhance their experience of doing investigative work, the teacher had planted crime scene clues in the park, including strategically placed individuals posing as dead bodies. But the students happened upon a body that to them seemed a little too dead. Imagine their surprise when they discovered it was the actual corpse of a homeless man who had died of natural causes. Without disturbing the body, how could they tell the difference between a real dead body and someone playing dead? The difference is energy. A living body has its vital force intact whereas a corpse does not.

The idea that living systems contain a vital force is not new. Vital energy has been recognized and actively worked with for thousands of years in various health systems. In traditional Chinese medicine the vital force plays a significant role. The energy channels flowing through the physical body are directly accessed by the careful placement of acupuncture needles. The needles act as tiny lightning rods attracting and redirecting the body's subtle energies. Acupressure, which utilizes the same channels without needles, also works with vital energy. Martial arts such as Kung Fu, Tai Chi, Qigong, Taekwondo, Karate, and Judo are all based in an understanding of the vital force. In Yoga and in Ayurveda, the Hindu science of life, energy is recognized as key to health. Across the spectrum from Tibetan medicine to Maori, Zulu, and Hawaiian healing methods energy plays a major role. In fact, in every indigenous system of medicine as well as in modern chiropractics, osteopathy, and homeopathy energy is a central concept.[7]

But when it comes to conventional Western medicine the energy aspect has been absent. If you go to the doctor and complain about feeling de-energized there is little to be done. Even when the situation becomes dire, as in the case of chronic fatigue, there is no treatment. Why has the vital force been overlooked? Most likely it's because Western medicine developed through the dissection and

study of cadavers. In other words, dead bodies. It's like examining
a matchstick whose flame is already extinguished versus one that
is actively burning. A dead body no longer has its vital force—its
interactive energy—intact. Conventional Western medicine offers a
highly sophisticated understanding of the physical components of
maladies but the energy aspect is missing.

Energy Comes From Energy

It is energy itself—not diet, sleep, or exercise—that gives you
energy. Energy comes from energy, flows into energy, and returns to
energy of differing forms. To focus our investigation, we'll look into
four basic energy bodies, one of which we've already mentioned.
The vital force, or vital body, is responsible for your vitality, your
"get-up-and-go" energy. The vital body animates you and brings
you to life. It carries the vital force that is responsible for your
overall health and your physical body's ability to heal. In fact, the
vital body is so intimately coupled with the physical body that they
must be understood together, as two aspects of the same body—a
vital/physical body. You are a living being, not a dead corpse. Your
vital body is intricately woven into your physical body. Despite that,
for convenience sake, I refer to the vital body and physical body as
though they are distinct, their dual aspect must be kept in mind:
they are two sides of the same coin.

Your vital body is responsible for the proper intake and
correct distribution of energy throughout your system. It is directly
linked to physical health as well as to mental functioning and
emotional wellbeing. In fact, your vital body is greatly affected
by thoughts and emotions. In turn, it affects your physical body
and provides the invisible link between your mind and your body.
The seamless connection of your mind and body can no longer be
denied. Although thoughts and feelings cannot be viewed under a
microscope, newly developed biotechnologies now track their effects
in the physical body. It's possible to watch a computer monitor
and actually see a person's brain and body change in response to

stressful thoughts or feelings. Thoughts and emotions themselves act as powerful energy forces.

It's well known that stress, meaning *distress*, is the great destroyer of health and wellbeing. It's the common denominator in all ten of the top deadly diseases. That's because stress drains vitality. It depletes energy in stealthy ways since virtually anything can produce stress. Even happy events, such as a work promotion or a marriage ceremony, can be stressful.

One approach to stress reduction is to remove the stressors. If your distress comes from job related issues, relationship conflict, or traffic congestion the solution is to quit the job, end the conflicted relationship, and drive at a different time. In other words, change the external conditions. But this potentially creates even more stress and often doesn't solve the problem. Anyone who has frequently switched jobs, altered schedules, or ended relationships realizes that we can change the externals but we take our problems with us. Often, the external approach is not really a solution but an attempted quick fix. It's only a matter of time before the old stressors creep in again or new ones take their place. Our control of the external environment is limited. Plus, *any* situation is a potential stressor.

It is energy itself that gives you energy.

On the way to work when traffic gets backed up, some people react by getting distressed but others don't. That means the stress is not out there in the traffic; it's inside the distressed person. By definition, stress is produced by an inability to adapt to change. Instead of adapting to a situation there is resistance. Thus, resistance is the true cause of stress. Your resistance or inability to adapt is determined by what goes on inside of you—what you are thinking and feeling at the time; your attitude toward the situation. Stress does not exist outside of you. Your reaction emerges out of your internal thoughts and feelings. Unlike the traffic, this is something you do have control over. The exercises in this book are designed to give you this kind of self-mastery.

In addition to vital energy, thoughts and feelings constitute two more types of energies we will investigate. Just as your vital body is responsible for your vitality, your emotional body is responsible for your feelings and your mental body for your thoughts. These energy bodies can be understood as distinct but overlapping channels of experience. Let's look at the simple act of drinking a glass of water. The physical aspect of drinking involves bodily processes. Your lips part to receive the glass, you taste the water as you swallow and feel it go down your esophagus. Your emotional experience refers to how you feel about it—sad, happy, anxious, grateful, etc. Then there are your thoughts; another simultaneous, yet distinct, aspect of your water-drinking experience. To put it all together, you can feel the physical sensation of the water going down while experiencing it as a happy thing and find yourself thinking about yesterday's rain shower that conveniently happened while you were inside a shop and then abruptly finished in time for you to get home completely dry. Your thoughts are distinguishable from your feelings, which are distinct from your bodily sensations; yet they all overlap.

So far we have accounted for your physical, emotional, and mental channels of experience. But there is something more. Although it's tempting to use the word *spiritual*, we'll avoid it. Too many people equate the spiritual with religion and we don't want to confuse the two. For lack of a better word, we'll use the term *universal* instead. If you think about it, any aspect of your internal experience can be seen as belonging to one of four arenas—the vital/physical, emotional, mental, or something beyond these (universal). You have four bodies in one.[8] Your physical, emotional, mental, and universal bodies constitute the equipment needed to function in life and your vital body is their power supply. The vital body is responsible for the energy needed to charge your other bodies.

Your four bodies are not separate. On the contrary, they are overlapping and quite interconnected. But rarely are these four parts of you in agreement. That's why it's sometimes difficult to make decisions and, once you make them, it can be hard to follow through. Each one of your bodies has an agenda of its own and can pull you in different directions, a big waste of energy. Each of the bodies is prone to certain conditions, which we will explore in depth, along with their solutions. The four bodies comprise your subtle energy make-up and are responsible for your overall energy health.

Energy is Inergy

Unfortunately, the word *energy* is confusing because it's used to refer to a wide variety of things. It tends to conjure up images of electricity, nuclear power, wind generators, and the like. The subtle energy we're concerned with has three distinct qualities that get missed by the generic term *energy*. Our energy is:

- Accessed *internally*

- Nonphysical *energy*

- Coupled with *information*

First, the energies of vitality, emotions, thoughts and so forth are found inside of you. Despite outward appearances or what you may display to the world, you—and only you—know what is going on inside of you at any given moment via the invisible energy bodies described above (vital, emotional, mental and universal). These subtle energy channels are unique to living humans. Machines cannot produce them. They are experienced subjectively, inside of you, and you have the capacity to be aware of them. Only you know what you are feeling, thinking and experiencing internally at any given moment.

Second, as already discussed, subtle energy is nonphysical.[9] This means it is essentially not electromagnetic (although it may show up this way in the physical body) nor is it the energy produced by the cell's mitochondria/ATP interaction mentioned at the start of this chapter. It is beyond the perceptible range of ordinary physics and does not necessarily abide by physical laws.

At the turn of the 20th Century when scientists probed deeply into physical matter to discover what we are truly made of, they were stunned to find that dense material substance consists of mostly empty space. Further investigation revealed that so-called "empty" space is not so empty. Quite the opposite of a vacuum, space is a dynamic and absolute fullness of luminous infinite energy.[10]

- In one cubic centimeter of empty space, there is energy greater than the total amount of energy embedded in all matter in the known universe

- Matter is actually space itself in a crystallized, condensed energy form

- Space is efflorescent, radiating and consisting of woven light

- At a very short distance (10 to the minus 33cm) space and time as we know it break down into a dynamic froth, called the *quantum foam*

- If you took all the mass in the visible universe and fused it together into pure energy, and then took all that energy and compressed it into 1 cubic centimeter, you'd still have to add about *14 more orders of magnitude* to even come close to the potency of this foam

- You are this energy

Since quantum physics has been around for over a century, its application to our functioning seems long overdue. We must come to understand ourselves according to what is now known about the true nature of reality: energy in various forms is the core of everything, including us.

Third, this energy is laced with information.[11] Sometimes called *enformy* or *active information*, subtle energy is intelligent, informed, and responsive. Thus, your bodily system is best understood as a communication system.[12] Subtle energy contains messages that impact us but often we don't know how to interpret them. It's as if we are living in a 3-D movie but we're not wearing the special glasses to really see what's going on. Because subtle energies are intimately coupled with information, they are meant to be interacted with. You can learn to encode and decode their messages. This book will teach you ways of doing that.

To help distinguish this type of subtle energy from other types of energy we'll use the term *inergy*, which translates as, *energy coupled with information and accessed inside* (energy + information + inside = inergy). It refers to the subtle energy/ information channels accessible inside you. To serve as a reminder of the unique qualities of this type of energy, from now on I will be using the term *inergy* instead of *energy*.

Let's try a simple exercise to give you a hands-on experience of this inergy. [12] The following exercise, like many in the remainder of the book, asks you to close your eyes and use your internal senses. This requires reading ahead in order to follow the instructions of the exercise. (To help free your hands and eyes from being tied to the book, go to www.EndlessEnergyBook.com for free audio downloads in which I facilitate many of the exercises.)

Exercise: Sensing Inergy

- Hold both of your hands in front of you, shoulder width apart with your palms facing up.

- Read ahead to the end of the exercise and then close your eyes to do the exercise. It's important to keep your eyes closed during the entire exercise because you are asked to feel and sense your hands but not look at them visually.

- Close your eyes and focus your awareness on your two hands. Pay particular attention to sensing the size of your hands. How do they feel? Does one hand feel larger or smaller than the other? Are they about the same size? If you're like most people, your two hands will feel very similar in size with your eyes closed.

- Then pick one of your hands; it doesn't matter which one. Keeping your eyes closed, focus your whole attention on the chosen hand. Send a clear message to the chosen hand that this hand is bigger than the other. Spend at least one full minute with focused attention sending that specific inergy (energy/information) to the chosen hand. Tell your chosen hand that it is much longer than your other hand. Visualize that your fingers are longer, your palm is wider, and your overall hand is larger. Again, take as least a minute to sincerely do this.

- Then, keeping your eyes closed, recheck the size of your hands by sensing the hands. Do they feel different? How do they compare? Does one hand feel larger or smaller than the other?

- When the comparison feels complete, you can open your eyes.

If you're like most people, you will sense an important difference in the size of your hands after completing the exercise. When you have your eyes closed, the hand that you focused on will feel considerably larger than the other. It's as if your chosen hand received the message and responded accordingly. But what about your physical hand? When you open your eyes you can see that your hand is not physically larger. Your eyes indicate that your hands are still the same size. So what difference does it make if you imagine your hand getting bigger? Or, put another way, what difference does it make if you use your intent to visualize your hand getting bigger and then sense it is so?

We know that we have five senses: vision, hearing, taste, touch, and smell. These senses extend out into the world and detect the sights, sounds, smells and stimuli of our external environment. What we are not told is that, in addition to those external senses, we also have internal senses. In the exercise above, five internal senses were used: attention, visualization, self-talk, self-sensing, and intent. These senses detect and influence the unseen world of inergies. When you focus your inergy/intent on your chosen hand to get bigger, believe it or not, the vital body of your chosen hand can actually respond by growing in size.[13] Your internal senses are inergy tools designed to detect and interact with the inergy aspects of your system.

There's a fundamental difference between external and internal senses. External senses help us orient to the material world, giving us information about the physical environment. Internal senses help us orient to the unseen world of inergies. Just as we rely on our external senses to guide us as we navigate through the physical world, our internal senses are necessary in the world of inergies. We'll learn more about your internal senses and four bodies (vital, emotional, mental, and universal) in the next chapter.

How to Use This Guide

If you want to have a fit and healthy physical body, you may join a gym and consult with a personal trainer. The trainer acts as a health guide, assessing your particular needs, teaching you about aspects of your body, training you in various fitness methods, and coaching you along the way so that you can achieve your overall health goals. Changing unhealthy habits can be difficult and many people don't stay the course. It requires support on the part of the trainer and commitment to change on the part of the participant. Although a training program can be sometimes arduous and challenging, the job of a trainer is to make it fun and exciting while achieving results.

If you'll allow me to act as your inergy trainer, I will guide you in a program to achieve optimal inergy health. The remainder of this book is organized as a training program for your four bodies. It starts with an assessment of your four bodies to find out their overall condition. Then we'll learn about each body individually, followed by exercises specific to that particular body. At the end, we'll bring the pieces back together and complete a final assessment. You may want to read the book through first to familiarize yourself with the program before engaging in the exercises. As your personal inergy health guide, I'll do my best to make the experience as enjoyable and easy as possible. Although we'll look at each of your bodies individually, this separation is done for the purpose of learning more about them. In day-to-day living, the bodies overlap and can be difficult to discern.

As with any training program, the approach used in this book is one of many. It is not meant to replace other resources but is meant to complement and be used in combination with them. Most importantly, the book does not make any claim that its contents are intended to treat or diagnose disease or psychiatric conditions. It does not advance or substitute for medical advice or psychotherapy. If you believe you have a physical, emotional, or mental health problem, please consult a health professional right away.

When you work with a coach and embark on a training program, you can enter at the beginning, intermediate or advanced level. The exercises described are organized according to level of difficulty, starting with beginners. Although it may be tempting to skip a level, the exercises build on each other, so it is advised that you start at the beginner level and advance from there. The same holds true for training each body. The chapters are arranged in sequential order—vital, emotional, mental, and universal—from lower to higher frequency with each chapter building on the previous. Although it's possible to skip around, some of the concepts and terms may not make sense out of order.

This book is not meant to be an exhaustive exploration of the inergy bodies. Rather, the intent is to present an introductory guide with enough basic information to get you started on an inergy health program. The field of energy medicine is emergent with new discoveries and modalities being readily developed. This information is a starting point, not the definitive source. Appendix A at the end of the book contains a list of some key organizations and websites. Stay tuned for more exciting advances! In the meantime, the next step is to get an overview of your four inergy bodies.

Chapter Two

Your Four Bodies

You've just arrived at a gathering at a friend's house. You're standing near the door talking with an acquaintance when suddenly you get the distinct impression that someone is staring at you. You can feel the eyes. You turn around to find out who it is. Sure enough, there is your ex on the other side of the room eying you. You finish your conversation and walk across the room to the food table. On your way you see your best friend from work but something tells you not to stop and talk. You get the sense that she is in a bad mood so you keep going. Just when you are about to pick up a plate and help yourself to some appetizers you encounter a stranger who seems warm and friendly. You strike up a conversation, making appropriate small talk. As you're conversing he keeps inching closer. When he gets within about 12 inches, you feel uncomfortable and step back. He steps forward. He is encroaching on your space and you can feel it. You have to step back again. Thankfully the conversation ends abruptly and you can eat in peace.

In this scenario a lot of information was communicated without sound, visual cues, or touch contact. The palpable feeling of being stared at, the vibration given off by someone in a bad mood, the encroachment on your personal space; most of us sense and respond to the unseen world of inergy (energy/information) constantly without fully realizing what we are doing. Although these kinds of experiences are commonplace—and we are often correct in our sensibilities[1]—conventional science has no explanation for how they happen. But when we bring the inergy bodies into the picture everything comes into focus. The mysteries are solved. That's because your inergy bodies extend beyond your physical body for several feet creating an invisible, sensitive, multi-layered field of energy and information around you (see Figure 2.1).

Your inergy field consists of four layers of concentric forms that include your vital, emotional, mental, and universal bodies.[2] It accounts for the "eyes at the back of your head," as well as your ability to sense other people's emotions and moods. It also accounts for a variety of experiences commonly referred to as *psychic* or *paranormal.* The different dimensions of your inergy constitution are called *bodies* because if you could actually see inergies, you would be able to see that they have a particular form. Just as your physical body has its unique size and shape, so do your inergy bodies.

To better understand your inergy makeup we need to start with what we know about energy at a basic level. Namely, Albert Einstein's famous equation: $E=mc^2$. You may have heard of this before, but what does it mean in terms of your day-to-day energy levels? With this simple equation Einstein proved the interrelationship between the world of energy and dense physical matter. The equation translates as: energy equals mass times the speed of light squared. In ordinary terms, it means that energy and matter are interchangeable. Put another way: matter is the concentration of energy. It means that, in essence, everything is energy of varying densities, vibrating at different speeds. Even material objects are an expression of energy.

The Energy Continuum

Everything exists on an energy continuum ranging from the dense physical on one end of the spectrum to the unseen "indefinable" on the other. When the vibration slows down enough, into an ultra-low range, energy solidifies into material substance and shows up on the physical plane. You can see it and touch it. When the energy vibrates fast enough, at an ultra-high frequency, the dense physical substance drops away and energy becomes invisible. Yet it is still present. Energy changes forms but at its essence, everything is energy. We could say there is nothing but energy (or inergy as we have been calling it).

A similar kind of transformation process happens when water is heated or cooled. When water molecules are slowed down in low temperatures, the liquid water densifies into rock solid ice. When heated, the molecules vibrate faster and the hard ice transforms into a more liquid form. If the water is heated enough,

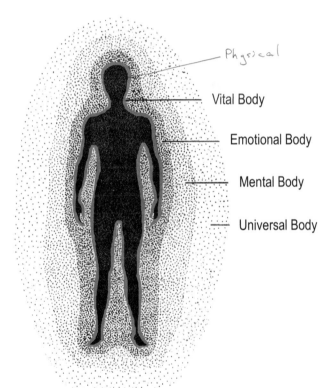

Physical

Vital Body

Emotional Body

Mental Body

Universal Body

Figure 2.1 The human inergy field with four layers:
the vital, emotional, mental, and universal bodies.

the molecules continue to vibrate even faster and the water turns into vaporized steam that eventually evaporates. Water occupies a continuum of dense physical ice (low vibration) on one end of the spectrum and moist air (high vibration) on the other. Although the water changes form, its essence is still water.

Similarly, everything exists on an inergy continuum with the lowest or slowest frequency, the world of solid substance, at one end of the spectrum. At the other end is fast/high frequency, ethereal vibration. Within these two extremes are several gradations. Each of us exists on this same continuum. Not only is everything inergy but *everyone* is inergy. At the lowest frequency end of the spectrum is your physical body. It comprises a relatively small fraction of your overall constitution. At the highest frequency end is your universal body. In between are your vital, emotional, and mental bodies.

Using words like *lowest* or *highest* is not meant to suggest that lower is worse and higher is better. Steam is not better than ice. It depends on what you want to use it for. *Lower* and *higher* may sound hierarchical but these are merely terms used to differentiate inergy frequencies. The higher levels are not more valuable than the lower. These words just provide a way to label two differing frequency bands. If, for example, we were talking about musical notes and I referred to high C and low C, that wouldn't mean that high C is better than low C, it just helps distinguish between the two.

You exist on a gradated continuum that ranges from ultra-low to ultra-high frequency inergy. This means you occupy multiple levels of experience simultaneously. The water lily has been used as an appropriate metaphor for understanding how this works. Just as the water lily takes root in a muddy lake bottom, you exist on the material plane with your vital/physical body. You have aspects extending beyond that (your emotional and mental bodies), much like the stem of the water lily extends up through the water forming a lily pad on the surface. When you develop your higher frequency aspects (universal body) you can fully blossom, just as the lily's flower transcends the water and blooms in the air and sunlight. Unlike other flowers, the water lily exists on four levels (earth, water, air, light) at the same time because it is equipped to experience these four distinct dimensions simultaneously. Similarly, you exist on four levels simultaneously (vital/physical, emotional, mental, and universal) because you are equipped with four bodies that enable you to do so.

If you are more technologically inclined, think about your inergy make-up in terms of a common household remote control. One button can turn on your television, one can activate your stereo, another can switch on your DVD player, and so forth. Each component's signal occupies a distinct frequency band. The signals emitted from the remote are invisible energy/information forces, yet they are all housed together in one unit, the physical hand-held remote control. When you press the television button only the television turns on or off, not the stereo or DVD. The signals are distinct but they also overlap because you can have all of the components—the TV, DVD and stereo—activated at once.

In terms of your inergy constitution, your physical body is akin to the remote control unit itself. Because everything is inergy, the physical remote control unit is also inergy, vibrating at an ultra-low frequency. Like the remote, your vital/physical body acts as a kind of receiver, or communication matrix, for the other frequencies.[3] Your other bodies are similar to the invisible signals of the remote. Just as the signals occupy distinct frequency bands, so do your inergy bodies.

The lowest vibrational form that your inergy constitution takes is the physical level of material substance; this is evident by the fact that you have a physical body. I won't go into detail about the physical body because this book is about the rest of your inergy components. Numerous books and resources are available that focus on physical health alone. In fact, Western medicine has been exclusively devoted to studying and repairing the dense physical body. But there is much more to you than that.

One of the things that make humans so complex is that we occupy multiple channels of experience simultaneously. To continue with the remote control metaphor, the frequency bands of the remote are not tied to a specific component, individual, or location. They are universal frequency channels that exist invisibly in the ethers, readily available to be used by anyone. You can buy a universal remote at a store and program it to work with any television or electronic component that will calibrate to a remote.

So it is with your inergy bodies. They represent your uniquely calibrated signals that exist within larger, universally available frequency bands (see Figure 2.2).[4] The frequency bands are like channels of experience. They consist of the vital, emotional, mental, and universal levels. The uniquely calibrated signal is called a *body* and is made up of a particular energy/information configuration. Essentially, your unique experiences on each of the corresponding channels of existence program your bodies. Thus, each body has a particular shape and condition.

To find out the current condition of your inergy bodies, we'll start with an assessment of each. Similar to an intake questionnaire and photo used by a personal trainer, this will give us a clearer picture of each of your inergy bodies to help assess their needs. It will also be used for "before and after" comparisons. (A copy of the assessment is provided at the end of the book in an Epilogue so you can retake it, if you choose, after you've had a chance to do some of the inergy exercises in the upcoming chapters.)

Your Internal Senses

To do the assessment you are asked to use your internal senses, a level of functioning you are constantly enacting but may not know by name. We have quite a few internal senses[5] but we will focus on six to begin with.

- Attention
- Intention
- Visualization
- Self-Talk
- Self-Sensing
- Self-Observation

Your Inergy Constitution and
the Four Main Channels of Experience

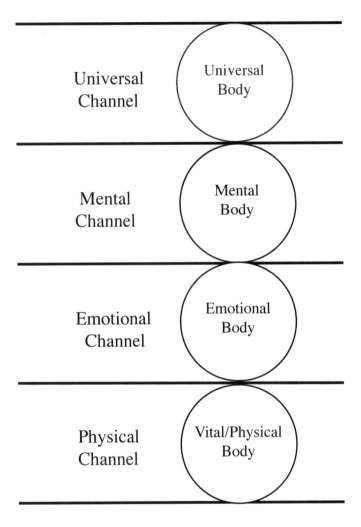

Figure 2.2 The four major channels of experience, also called the *planes of existence*, and the four inergy bodies that are formed upon those channels.

These senses are valuable internal resources. Just as the external senses of, say, seeing and hearing are vital to physical health, your internal senses are essential to your inergy health.

Attention

Inergy is responsive to attention. When you pay attention to something, you focus your external and internal senses on it. Your attention is like a spotlight that illuminates and brings to life that which it is directed upon. Simply put, inergy follows attention. Your attention in and of itself has potency.[6] What you focus your attention on receives inergy and is changed at a fundamental level. Sometimes called the *observer effect*, the idea is that the very act of observing something alters it in some way.

This surprising aspect of reality was first touched on by Nobel Prize winning physicist Werner Heisenberg when he published the mathematics of the Uncertainty Principle around 1926. The notion was further substantiated by the Copenhagen Interpretation in which an unobserved object is said to exist as potential until the observer chooses what to observe. The mere act of observation, of bringing your attention to something, inevitably changes it. Your attention is a transformative inergetic tool. We will discuss more about how this works in Chapter 9.

Intention

If attention is like a spotlight then intention is like a laser beam. Intention is attention infused with will (another internal sense). You are not just paying attention to something, you are willfully desiring a particular outcome. Inergy is extremely responsive to intent.[7] Intent can be used to mobilize your own inergy and to direct inergies to any place you choose at any time.

In Sao Paulo, Brazil, on June 3, 1998, three healers were directing healing intention to five volunteers who were over 6000 miles away in a research lab in Las Vegas, Nevada.[8] The five volunteers were hooked up to various monitoring devices to measure their heart rates, blood volume, breathing, and skin activity. At the exact timed intervals that the healers were sending their healing intent, the volunteers were registering the effects with monitor lights blinking and gauges fluctuating. During intervals when there was no intent, there were no effects, a clear demonstration of the precise power of intent.

Experiments such as this and hundreds of others confirm the effects of human intent on everything from fellow humans, to animals, insects, plants, bacteria, yeasts, cancer cells, and DNA.[9] We will discuss more about how this works in Chapter 7.

Visualization

Visualization is the capacity to use your mind to form concepts. We all have this ability but some have developed it more than others. Unlike the name suggests visualization is not limited to the visual realm. Probably a better term would be *sensualization*, because more than just the visual sense is potentially involved. Some people orient visually and are able to conjure up clear, vivid mental pictures or movies. Some who are more auditory think in terms of sounds or words. Others, more kinesthetic, will experience bodily sensations and feelings, a felt-sense about something. Additional orientations include mathematical, spatial, and musical. Ideally, we would want to employ as many senses as possible. Still, the three primary processes are visual, auditory and kinesthetic, with one of the three typically more predominant. When I use the word *visualization* I am including the other orientations as well, not just the visual.

Visualization, or guided imagery, is a potent tool for mobilizing inergies that is often successfully used by athletes to improve performance.[10] In one simple study participants were divided into three groups. One group was asked to go to a nearby gym every day for 20 minutes and practice making basketball free throws. A second group was asked to stay home and simply visualize completing successful free throws for 20 minutes each day. The third group, the control group, did nothing. After a month there was only one percent difference in the achievement level of those who actually practiced free throws at the gym (24% improvement) versus those who stayed home and visualized (23% improvement). The control group showed no change. This experiment and others like it have been repeated with consistent results.

Visualization is imagination with intent. It is not day dreaming, brainstorming, or stream of consciousness thinking. It is not about opening your mind up to see what floats in. Visualization is purposeful imagining that involves holding a specific focus through the power of concentration. When you focus your sense of smell on a fragrant flower, for example, the invisible scent molecules waft toward your nose so you can take them in. Similarly, when you use your internal sense of visualization to focus on something, you attract corresponding inergies from the surroundings to bring the changes you desire into existence. The more clear your concentration, the stronger your results. We will learn more about the mechanisms of this in Chapter 7.

Self-Talk

Just as we all visualize, we all talk to ourselves. Researchers refer to this as *explanatory style*, but most of us know it as the "tapes" playing inside our heads, the noisy mind, or the inner critic. Self-talk constitutes the messages you tell yourself about what you experience and it has profound effects on your health.[11] None of us perceives reality in its pure form. It is always subject to personal interpretation. The meaning you give to what you perceive, how you view it, what you feel about it, the pictures you envision, the words and phrases you tell yourself—this is your self-talk. Such internal dialogue may take various forms but it still qualifies as self-talk. For some people it's more visual, for others more verbal, or even a felt-sense.

If you have visual self-talk you likely see pictures and images in your head, as if you are playing an internal movie that parallels your life experience. A person whose self-talk is more sensate will tend to feel subtle internal impressions and physical sensations in response to life. If your self-talk is verbal, you probably have a running commentary going on. Your experience of the world would be primarily processed through words and sounds. You may also have a combination of these. The point is, we do interact with ourselves internally. We encourage, nag, inform, criticize, support and entertain ourselves through an inner channel of expression. This is the internal sense of self-talk.

Self-Sensing

While self-talk represents a relatively narrow channel of communication, you also have the capacity to expand your focus to fill your entire body. This is self-sensing. While self-talk is primarily a channel of internal expression, self-sensing is a mode of internal listening. It is an inner-focused, subjective stance of experiencing yourself from the "inside-out." It occurs by shifting your attention away from an external focus and directing your attention toward an internal focus, then broadening your focus to include your whole body. Self-sensing can be used to sense into a selected organ, such as your lungs or liver. It can also be used to sense pain or to apprehend more subtle internal sensations. Because inergy follows attention, bringing your attention inside your body via self-sensing has proven therapeutic effects.[12] It allows you to experience a vast array of internal functioning including bodily sensations, feelings, thoughts, intentions, insights, dreams, imaginings, and so forth. It is a broad channel of internal receptivity that opens you up to a variety of inergies.

Self-Observation

Self-observation refers to the ability to observe what is going on inside of you. It includes the array of internal functioning mentioned above and may sound identical to self-sensing. However, there is a fundamental difference between the two. With self-sensing, you are actually *experiencing* the multitude—or specifically selected—internal functioning that you are focused upon. You are actively engaged with your inner landscape. In contrast, with self-observation you are *observing* it in a more detached way. You are witnessing or watching what is going on inside of you, spectating, as it were, instead of actively participating. Sometimes this practice is called *mindfulness*. We will discover more about the importance of self-observation in Chapter 7.

Before and After Assessment

Now that you have a basic understanding of your internal senses, let's return to our Before and After assessment. Starting with your vital body, we'll look into the condition of each body through a series of simple questions. Keep the results of your inventory in a place where you can refer back to them as a useful reference for the remainder of the book in which we explore each of your bodies individually. The book ends with a re-take of the assessment in the Epilogue.

Your Vital Body

The four part Before and After assessment begins with your vital body, which requires a brief overview to help you complete the first step. We'll explore this body in more detail in the next chapter. Your vital body is woven into your physical body and extends beyond it for several inches. It constitutes your power-supply, responsible for distributing life-force inergy throughout your system. When your vital body is healthy you have stamina and feel invigorated. You glow, radiating health and vitality. When your vital body is depleted, you feel de-energized and lethargic. Much effort is required to move through your day, as if you were somehow swimming against life's current.

Although the condition of your vital body may fluctuate throughout the day, the intention here is to get a general idea of it. Using the following exercise as a guide, answer the questions keeping in mind the overall condition of your vital body.

Exercise: Vital Body Assessment

- Find a quiet place in which you can focus without distraction.

- Be in a seated position, as comfortable as possible.

- Take a couple of slow, deep breaths.

- Gently close your eyes and intentionally shift your attention away from an external focus toward an internal focus, awakening your internal senses.

- Once you have made this shift, again using the power of your intent, consciously focus your attention on your vital body to the best of your ability. Using self-talk, tell yourself that you are now focusing on your vital body.

- Do your best to sense into your vitality, the substance of your vital body, using your capacity to self-sense. How does it feel? What is your vitality level? Energized or depleted? Focus your attention specifically on your vital body and allow yourself to get a palpable experience of it to the best of your ability. There is no right or wrong, just use an attitude of curiosity.

- Then shift to a self-observer mode, where you are looking at your vital body instead of experiencing it. Like a detached detective, examine your vital body, noticing everything you can about it.

- Ask yourself the following questions and jot down your answers on a sheet of paper.

- Spend 15-30 seconds with each question. If nothing comes up as you ask the question, leave it blank and move on to the next.

  - What does your vital body look like?

  - How big is it?

  - What color is it?

  - What shape is it?

  - How does it move?

  - What does it sound like?

  - What does it feel like?

  - If your vital body could speak, what would it say?

  - What is the overall condition of your vital body?

- Take a moment to draw a simple sketch of your vital body.

Your Emotional Body

Although your vital body plays an important role in your health and wellbeing, there is much more to you than that. In addition to having vitality and the power to move, you also have the capacity to experience emotions. Just as your physical body has its unique shape, so does your emotional body. It is formed by your experiences on the emotional plane. This channel of experience is quite vast and alluring with many tantalizing adventures available. The deepest, darkest lows to the most ecstatic highs—and everything in between—can be found on the emotional channel.

We know that colds and flu get passed around on the physical level but emotions, too, are extremely contagious. In fact, research shows that within two minutes of being in the same room with someone who is experiencing a strong emotion—pleasant or unpleasant—you pick up on the emotion and begin to experience it yourself.[13] In a vivid example of how invisible inergies affect us, it doesn't matter what you've previously been feeling and it doesn't even matter if the person is a loved one or a complete stranger. This phenomenon is referred to as *emotional contagion.*[14]

Since many of us have unhealthy emotional bodies, it's easy to contract inergetic pathogens and pass them around like a social virus. Fear and anger seem to have reached epidemic proportions, but there is no "vaccine." If you practice the exercises in this book, however, you can do a lot to boost your emotional body's immune system. We'll look further into your emotional body in Chapter 5.

Use the following exercise as a guide to assess the overall condition of your emotional body.

Exercise: Emotional Body Assessment

- Find a quiet place in which you can focus without distraction.

- Be in a seated position, as comfortable as possible.

- Take a couple of slow, deep breaths.

- Gently close your eyes and intentionally shift your attention away from an external focus toward an internal focus, awakening your internal senses.

- Once you have made this shift, again using the power of your intent, consciously focus your attention on your emotional body to the best of your ability.

  Using self-talk, tell yourself you are now focusing on your emotional body.

- Do your best to sense into your feelings, the substance of your emotional body, using your capacity to self-sense. How does it feel? What is your emotional landscape like? Are you feeling irritated, disappointed, anxious, glad? Focus your attention specifically on your emotional body and allow yourself to get a palpable experience of it to the best of your ability. There is no right or wrong, just use an attitude of curiosity.

- Then shift to a self-observer mode, where you are looking at your emotional body instead of experiencing it. Like a detached detective, examine your emotional body, noticing everything you can about it.

- Ask yourself the following questions and jot down your answers on a sheet of paper.

- Spend 15-30 seconds with each question. If nothing comes up as you ask the question, leave it blank and move on to the next.

  - What does your emotional body look like?

  - How big is it?

  - What color is it?

  - What shape is it?

  - How does it move?

  - What does it sound like?

  - What does it feel like?

- If your emotional body could speak, what would it say?

- What is the overall condition of your emotional body?

- Take a moment to draw a sketch of your emotional body.

Your Mental Body

Your mental body is probably very familiar to you since most of our educational system is focused on developing it. Your mental body gives you the capacity to think thoughts, which is a frequency channel distinct from the emotional or vital. Concerned with facts, linear logic, reasoning, and opinions, it allows you to analyze and synthesize information. When you are engaged in problem-solving and trying to figure things out, you are exercising your mental body.

Your mental body also is capable of self-awareness and self-monitoring. A highly developed mental body has the power of concentration and capacity to hold a focus. It is concerned with wisdom and truths in addition to knowledge and facts. It can be used for thinking about the bigger picture and gaining insights. The mental body allows you to see behind things, to see the essence of things, and "connect the dots" of your experience. Because of its close proximity to your emotional body, your mental body can be heavily influenced by emotional concerns. We'll explore your mental body further in Chapter 7.

Use the following exercise as a guide to assess the overall condition of your mental body.

Exercise: Mental Body Assessment

- Find a quiet place in which you can focus without distraction.

- Be in a seated position, as comfortable as possible.

- Take a couple of slow, deep breaths.

- Gently close your eyes and intentionally shift your attention away from an external focus toward an internal focus, awakening your internal senses.

- Once you have made this shift, again using the power of your intent, consciously focus your attention on your mental body to the best of your ability. Using self-talk, tell yourself that you are now focusing on your mental body.

- Do your best to sense into your thoughts, the substance of your mental body, using your capacity to self-sense. What kind of thoughts are there? What is your mental landscape like? Is it slow, spacious or quiet? Fast, noisy or crowded? Focus your attention specifically on your mental body and allow yourself to get a palpable experience of it to the best of your ability. There is no right or wrong, just use an attitude of curiosity.

- Then shift to a self-observer mode, where you are looking at your mental body instead of experiencing it. Like a detached detective, examine your mental body, noticing everything you can about it.

- Ask yourself the following questions and jot down your answers on a sheet of paper.

- Spend 15-30 seconds with each question. If nothing comes up as you ask the question, leave it blank and move on to the next.

  - What does your mental body look like?

  - How big is it?

  - What color is it?

  - What shape is it?

  - How does it move?

  - What does it sound like?

  - What does it feel like?

  - If your mental body could speak, what would it say?

  - What is the overall condition of your mental body?

- Take a moment to draw a sketch of your mental body.

Your Universal Body

In addition to your physical, emotional, and mental bodies you have a universal body. This body is concerned with awareness that is beyond the intellect, beyond the mind as we know it. It is associated with intuitive insights, right use of will, unity consciousness, and beingness itself. These may be hard concepts to grasp at first, especially since they are difficult to describe in words. It may be helpful to think about your universal body as occupying the space in between your thoughts and feelings. Since your actions, thoughts and emotions are always changing, can they be who you are? When you are *not* thinking, doing, or feeling, you are still here, so there must be something more to you.

When physicists were splitting atoms over a hundred years ago to find the core of our existence, they discovered that, at its essence, matter is not fixed. It is open-ended energy. It is no-thing. Your universal body is no-thing: it is not physical substance, action, emotion or thought. We could say it is closer to the essence of who you are since you are not your physical body, actions, emotions, or thoughts. You are the one who initiates the actions, experiences the emotions, thinks the thoughts. These things come and go but you—the universal you—remain constant. To refer back to the remote control metaphor, the universal body is the operator of the remote, the one pressing the buttons and doing the channel surfing. For now, we just want to get a glimpse of your universal body. We will explore it in more depth in Chapter 9.

Use the following exercise as a guide to assess the overall condition of your universal body.

Exercise: Universal Body Assessment

- Find a quiet place in which you can focus without distraction.

- Be in a seated position, as comfortable as possible.

- Take a couple of slow, deep breaths.

- Gently close your eyes and intentionally shift your attention away from an external focus toward an internal focus, awakening your internal senses.

- Once you have made this shift, again using the power of your intent, consciously focus your attention on your universal body to the best of your ability. Using self-talk, tell yourself that you are now focusing on your universal body.

- Do your best to sense into the space between your thoughts and feelings, the substance of your universal body, using your capacity to self-sense. How do you experience it? What is your universal landscape like? Can you be in the no-thingness? Focus your attention specifically on your universal body and allow yourself to get a palpable experience of it to the best of your ability. There is no right or wrong, just use an attitude of curiosity.

- Then shift to a self-observer mode, in which you look at your universal body instead of experiencing it. Like a detached detective, examine your universal body, noticing everything you can about it.

- Ask yourself the following questions and jot down your answers on a sheet of paper.

- Spend 15-30 seconds with each question. If nothing comes up as you ask the question, leave it blank and move on to the next.

  - What does your universal body look like?

  - How big is it?

  - What color is it?

  - What shape is it?

  - How does it move?

  - What does it sound like?

- What does it feel like?

- If your universal body could speak, what would it say?

- What is the overall condition of your universal body?

- Take a moment to draw a sketch of your universal body.

The vital/physical, emotional, mental and universal bodies make up your inergy constitution. They represent gradations of inergy on a continuum that ranges from ultra-low frequency dense physical matter at one end, to extreme-high frequency universal inergies at the other. Our four bodies give us four different channels of experience. But sometimes we limit ourselves to only a few channels. It's as if we own a four-story penthouse with a great view but we end up hanging out in the parking garage. We do not utilize all that is available to us.

When you look at the assessments of your bodies together you can get a sense of your overall inergy health. How do your bodies compare? You may find that one or more of your bodies is underweight and neglected. Conversely, you may also find that a particular body is demanding all of your attention. It may be overweight or over-trained. Ideally, we want all of the bodies to be fit, healthy, and working cooperatively together. The next step toward this goal is to take a look at each of your bodies individually, starting with your vital body.

Chapter Three

Your Vital Body

In training for World War II, Richard Morrison was a young naval officer aboard the USS *Wyoming*. An exemplary serviceman, Richard excelled in the various aspects of military life. One day during an emergency training maneuver he was required to abandon ship, board a transport boat, jump over the side of the boat, and bolt toward a target on the beach. Richard completed the drill with his customary precision and speed. It wasn't until after he reached the target and began to catch his breath that he looked down and noticed his left finger was missing. Later it was determined that in thrusting himself over the side of the boat his wedding ring had caught on the rail. The momentum of his thrust pulled his finger out, including a good part of the tendon.

After the incident Richard continued to feel sensations in his missing finger, as if it were still there. He expected these would go away when his body had a chance to heal and the hole that was left between his fingers completely closed. But that didn't happen. He continued to feel heat, cold, and sometimes the missing finger would itch, an itch that Richard could never satisfy. He didn't understand and wanted the phantom sensations to stop but they never did. Instead they got worse. As time went by, the missing finger began to throb with pain. Thinking it a little crazy, Richard took aspirin to try to help it, but to no avail. The pain persisted. The doctors said there was nothing to be done about it. How can you treat a finger that isn't there?

Richard wasn't alone. About 80% of amputees experience some kind of discomfort in their missing limbs. Sensations of shooting pain or electric shocks are common. Some experience their missing limbs curled up in strangely contorted positions. Others feel their fingers clenched, painfully digging into their palms. Even the slightest movement in a nearby area can sometimes cause excruciating pain in the missing appendage. This phenomenon, documented in medical books since the 1700s, is referred to as *phantom pain.* To this day, modern medicine has no explanation for it.

Enter the vital body. The vital body is woven into the physical body and extends beyond it for several inches.[1] It powers the physical body through a complex network of inergy (energy/information) lines that flow throughout the physical layer. Phantom pain and phantom limb sensations are easily understood once the vital body is brought into the picture. Every appendage of the physical body has a vital body counterpart, known as etheric body parts. Even though Richard's physical finger was missing, his etheric finger was still intact, carrying inergy messages of sensation and movement to his brain. Despite the loss of its physical replica, the vital body continues to interface with the world, relaying its energy/information content back to the body system.[2]

The Interface Effect

In addition to being as exact replica of your physical body, your vital body acts as an interface between your physical body and your other inergy bodies. In the clothing world an interface performs important functions. It's most commonly used in the collar of a men's dress shirt to make the collar stiff so it can stand up. The purpose of an interface is to reinforce or add substance to whatever it is sewn into. It is usually stitched onto the inside of an out-facing piece of fabric. This makes it invisible when the garment is completed because the interface is concealed between layers of fabric.

So it is with the vital body. It reinforces the physical layer, adding inergetic substance to it. The vital body is primarily woven onto the inside of your physical body and is "invisible" from the outside. As an interface, the vital body reinforces the physical body, providing the inergy scaffolding upon which the physical body is built. Like a collar without an interface, if the physical body were without its vital body "backing," it would be limp and inanimate, unable to stand up.

Interfaces go between layers of fabric. Similarly, the vital body goes between the physical and the three remaining bodies— the emotional, mental and universal, creating reciprocity between them. Any of the bodies can be accessed through the vital body. This is why healing modalities that specifically involve the vital body (such as Classical Homeopathy, Acupuncture, Reiki, Therapeutic Touch, Emotional Freedom Technique, Touch for Health and other kinesiologies, to name a few) help with physical ailments as well as emotional and psychological issues. Similarly, the higher frequency inergies of your emotional, mental, and universal bodies heavily influence your vital inergy, which, in turn, impacts your physical body. Your vital body interfaces with and acts as a gateway to your other bodies.

The Anatomy of Your Vital Body

A complete science of inergy anatomy is found in health systems from cultures that devoted thousands of years to studying and working directly with the vital body. It's impossible to do justice in one chapter to all that is known about this body. This cannot be stressed enough. I have condensed a vast amount of information and over-simplified to give a very basic understanding, enough to provide a working knowledge for energy health purposes. In similar fashion, few of us know the mechanisms behind our physical body functioning, yet we attend to it every day.

Independent research done mostly in India and China contains a storehouse of wisdom about the inner workings of the vital body. In India vital energy is called *prana*. In China it is referred to as *chi*. The discoveries of long ago, upon which entire successful medical systems were built, are being increasingly validated by Western scientific methods.[3] Although the US medical world has been resistant to recognizing the vital body, mainstream culture has embraced its ancient methods. You don't have to look far today to see the popularity of yoga, acupuncture, and the martial arts. These practices emerged from cultures dedicated to complex and systematic study of the vital body (see Figure 3.1). When combining their contributions a comprehensive, detailed picture of human inergy anatomy is formed.

Your vital body interpenetrates and powers your physical body through a sophisticated network of inergy centers and distribution lines that branch into smaller and smaller inergy capillaries. The lines are called *meridians* in Chinese medicine and have been validated by a number of methods, including MRI.[4] The centers are often referred to as *chakra*, a Sanskrit word that means *round* or *wheel*. These, as well, have been experimentally verified.[5] Those who are able to see inergies have described these centers as looking like spinning wheels or vortices that range in size from about two inches in diameter to several inches, depending on their stage of development.[6] It's likely the ancients had the capacity to see these wheel-like inergy centers and named them accordingly. As evidence of the Interface Effect, the centers and meridians have been empirically linked to physical, emotional, and mental health.

The centers are like electrical power plants where high voltage inergy is transformed and distributed through a convergence of power lines. Your vital body interfaces with your physical body through these power distribution lines. This inergy network corresponds to your physical nervous system. When several of these "power lines" intersect, which happens at the major nerve centers in your body, they become even more potent.

There are seven places in your body where multiple lines cross over, forming a major power center. These centers are positioned at the intersection of 21 power lines, which represents a

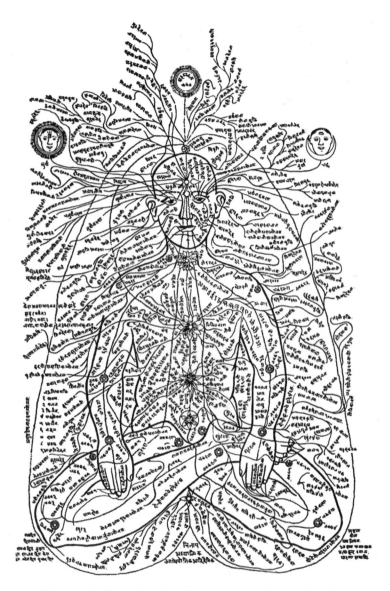

Figure 3.1 Chart depicting the complex understanding of
the human energy system from circa 19th Century Tibet
(attributed to the prophet Ratnasara).

high concentration of inergy. The seven major centers focalize into inergy channels that, in turn, feed into smaller centers, 21 minor and 49 mini centers.[7] The minor centers occur where 14 lines cross over and the mini centers are located where seven lines converge.

- 21 lines intersect = 7 major centers
- 14 lines intersect = 21 minor centers
- 7 lines intersect = 49 mini centers

The seven centers correspond to the major nerve plexus and endocrine glands of your physical body (see Figure 3.2).[8] The centers are funnel shaped. With the exception of the crown and base, the major centers have a smaller receiving end on the back of the body and a wider distribution end on the front. The centers are named for their corresponding locations in the physical body. Approximate locations are:

- Crown Center – The top of your head
- Brow Center – Your forehead
- Throat Center – Your throat
- Heart Center – The middle of your chest
- Solar Plexus Center – Your solar plexus
- Sacral Center – Your lower torso
- Base Center – The base of your spine

The centers supply the inergy necessary for optimal functioning of the organs, glands and nerves nearby their locations. The seven major centers govern specific physical aspects:[9]

- Crown – Right eye, upper brain, pineal gland
- Brow – Left eye, lower brain, pituitary gland
- Throat – Vocal apparatus, lungs, alimentary canal, thyroid, parathyroid
- Heart – Heart, circulation, blood, vagus nerve, thymus gland, immune system

The Seven Major Centers and
Corresponding Nerve Plexus

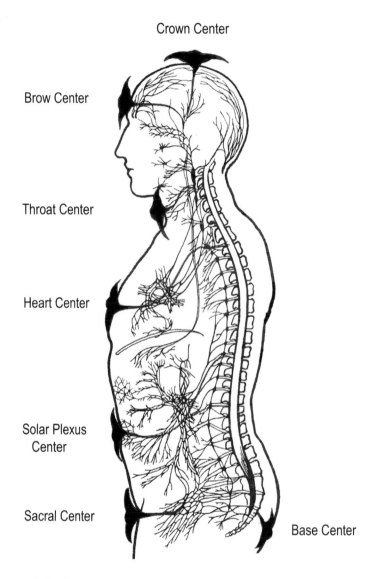

Figure 3.2 The seven major inergy centers shown with their corresponding anatomical nerve plexus and ganglia.

- Solar Plexus – Stomach, liver, gall bladder, pancreas, intestines, nervous system
- Sacral – Sex organs, reproductive system
- Base – Hips, kidneys, adrenal glands, spinal column

Although these seven centers are at various phases of development, all seven are functioning to a certain degree at all times. They play such a vital role in bringing life-sustaining inergy to the physical organs that without even one of them we cannot survive. The seven major centers never close down but they are at varying stages of health, most of which are determined by the condition of your emotional, mental, and universal bodies.

It may be tempting to focus attention and inergy into the centers to try to enhance them, as an increasing number of modalities facilitate (i.e., certain yoga, meditation, or breathing practices). However, this can negatively affect their delicate balance.[10] Due to the Interface Effect, the condition of the centers is largely determined by your psycho-emotional states. The best way to enhance a center is through conditioning your emotional and mental bodies.

The 21 minor centers are positioned throughout your body but are especially concentrated in your digestive areas, on your chest, and on your head. There are also minor centers in the palm of each hand, on the bottom of each foot, at the gonads, and at each knee. These minor centers along with their corresponding lines-of-force cause a concentration of inergy at these locations.

The centers and their power lines form an invisible network of inergies that flow throughout your physical body in a complex and intricate distribution system. Inergy flows into lines of ever decreasing size. There are 14 major lines of force that feed into about 200-400 smaller lines. These lines, in turn, branch out into tiny thread-like inergy capillaries, called *nadis*. Your vital body is comprised of approximately 72,000 of these.[11] To borrow a term from Star Trek, you are not a carbon unit. You are, in fact, a living, moving inergy being!

The Physiology of Your Vital Body

Physiology involves studying the functions and processes of organ systems. The physiology of your vital body is not tied to physical counterparts. It functions largely through the other bodies. The quest to understand the vital body took researchers straight into the emotional, mental, and universal bodies (the Interface Effect). The intimate relationship between the centers and the other bodies is such that each of the seven major centers is shown to be associated with particular psycho-emotional qualities. Again it must be stressed that I am oversimplifying; more thorough descriptions are available elsewhere.[12]

- Crown – Unity consciousness, selfless service
- Brow – Integration, insight, synthesis
- Throat – Conscious creativity, expression, intellect
- Heart – Compassion, understanding, forgiveness
- Solar Plexus – Emotions and desires
- Sacral – Boundaries
- Base – Will to survive

The crown center at the top of your head is associated with a kind of unity consciousness, a state of mind in which you see the interconnectedness of all. The ability to comprehend this wholeness brings about a desire to be of help to humanity. A developed crown center innately inspires you to some kind of service activity to help others. The more developed the crown, the wider your sphere of influence. In contrast, a person whose crown center is undeveloped will not find motivation in helping others. A moderately healthy crown center may produce a vague sense of a service calling that as yet cannot be acted on.

The next center, the brow, is connected with integration and intuitive insight.[13] This center provides the inergy necessary to help us see beyond opposites. A person who has a well-developed brow center will not get stuck in black-and-white thinking. Rather than seeing only two options (i.e., me versus you, big picture versus details, etc.) a developed brow center enables us to see the extremes as well as the many gradations in between and apply this capacity to any given situation. Instead of an *either/or* perspective there is one of synthesis and integration, *both/and.*

The throat center, which governs the whole vocal and breathing apparatus, takes something as subtle as breath and turns it into articulate verbal expression. The inergy of this center gives the capacity to take abstract ideas and turn them into a coherent plan of action. The throat center is at play when we are using our intellect. When it's healthy, we think clearly and creatively, accompanied by clarity in speech. When it's unhealthy, thinking is confused, communication muddled, and we can get stuck in a seemingly endless loop of trying to figure things out.

The heart center, as you might imagine, is connected with love, compassion, understanding, and forgiveness. When the heart center is developed, these qualities come easily with just about everyone we encounter. There is an overriding attitude of inclusion and connection. When it is underdeveloped, we are not capable of enacting this, or at least not very consistently. At times the function of the heart center is confused with emotional qualities. We are fond of saying: *My heart is heavy; my heart is happy,* or, *my heart is telling me not to do this.* However, the inergy of the heart is associated with pure love. It does not involve itself with emotional states such as trepidation, happiness, or fear. These kinds of emotions are the domain of the next lower center, at the solar plexus.

The solar plexus is considered the seat of emotions and desires. Inergetically speaking, emotion and desire are closely related. If you desire something (or someone, or a particular outcome to a situation), you are easily emotional about it. The pursuit of it can involve anxiety, titillation, and anticipation. If you get what you want, there is usually a rush of excitement and thrill or perhaps a sense of happiness. If you don't get what you want, the accompanying disappointment, hurt, regret, or resentment are usually not far away. Emotions can be highly motivational and inspirational, or they can be detrimental, depending upon what you do with them. An unhealthy solar plexus center can result if you habitually suppress or over-indulge your emotions (this will be discussed in Chapter 5).

The next center, the sacral center, governs the sexual organs and has to do with boundaries. Nowhere else do we lose our boundaries more than in the sex act. It is sometimes impossible to tell where you end or your partner begins. The lines get blurred. An unhealthy sacral center predicts boundary problems. A person can either have too loose or too rigid boundaries. A lack of boundaries can result in being overly available, say, sexually, emotionally, or physically (i.e., doing too much for everyone). Having boundaries that are too rigid results in the opposite. A person can be walled up emotionally, shutdown sexually, or live a very isolated life. It's also possible to have both—too rigid in some arenas and too loose in others.

The center at the base of the spine governs the hips, spine, kidneys and adrenals. This is the inergy of fight, flight or freeze and, appropriately, this center is associated with survival instincts. When it is healthy, the base of spine inergy gets activated only in dire circumstances when a survival reaction is called for. When it is unhealthy, everyday situations can evoke an alarm response. Say you lose some money in the stock market and react as if it's a life or death situation, or you misplace your cell phone and come undone. Maybe a date stands you up and it's the end of the world as you know it. These are signs of an unhealthy base of spine center. When the center is healthy, a survival reaction happens only in actual life-threatening situations.

If you find that you have identified with any of the unhealthy conditions touched on above, the inergy health approach is to address the condition at the level of your other inergy bodies. Because the vital body interfaces with the emotional, mental, and universal bodies via the centers, the key to healthy centers lies in the care of those bodies, what the remainder of this book is about.

The Top-Down Approach of Inergy Health

Within the paradigm of Western medicine most ailments, whether they are physical, emotional, or psychological, are often addressed from the bottom up, meaning, the physical level is the starting point. Health problems are typically treated with medications, tests, and surgeries that affect the physical body. Even emotional and psychological problems are increasingly treated with medications that alter physical body functioning. In contrast, the inergy health paradigm uses a top-down approach. Ailments are understood and addressed in terms of their next higher frequency level. As mentioned earlier, if there is indication of an unhealthy inergy center, go to the next higher level—the emotional—to remedy it. For an emotional issue, address the mental level, and so forth. The same holds true for the physical body. In the case of a physical problem, look to the vital body and its corresponding centers for a possible solution.

Each of the seven major centers has physical and psycho-emotional aspects:[14]

Physical	Center	Organ Systems	Psycho-Emotional Aspects
Head-top	Crown	Right eye; upper brain; pineal gland	Unity consciousness; selfless service
Forehead	Brow	Left eye; lower brain; pituitary gland	Integration; intuitive insight
Throat	Throat	Vocal apparatus; lungs; alimentary canal; thyroid	Conscious creativity; intellect; speech
Heart	Heart	Heart; blood; vagus nerve; thymus; immune system	Compassion; love; forgiveness
Solar Plexus	Solar Plexus	Digestive organs and nervous system	Emotions and desires
Sacrum	Sacral	Sex organs and reproductive system	Boundary concerns
Spine-base	Base	Hips; kidneys; adrenals; spinal column	Survival concerns

This allows you to go behind-the-scenes to unravel a physical symptom at the inergy level. You can do this by identifying the center closest to the location of your physical ailment and then looking at its psycho-emotional dimensions.

Let's say you have a hoarse voice that doesn't seem to respond to other treatments. On the physical level we can see the throat center governs the vocal apparatus, lungs, alimentary canal, and thyroid. On the psycho-emotional level the throat center has to do with the intellect, conscious creativity, and clear articulation thereof. To help solve the problem at the inergy level you can look into how you are dealing with your intellect. Are you under-utilizing your mind? Are you stuck in confusion or over-analysis? Are you being closed minded? Are you trying to figure something out that cannot be dealt with on the intellectual level? Are you ignoring your intuition? The answers to these questions can give clues to resolving your hoarse voice at the inergy level. The physical hoarseness is the effect while the emotional and mental bodies hold the key to the true cause. Although this example is an over-simplification, hopefully it gives you an idea of how to understand physical effects in terms of their underlying inergies.

The Blueprint Effect

We have been told that genes are the blueprint for our physical body. However, groundbreaking research in molecular biology over the last couple of decades has upset the conventional wisdom. Although genes play a fundamental role in determining our physicality, the new field of epigenetics (*epigenetic* means *above the gene*) has revealed another influence beyond our genes that determines whether or not a gene is used.

More like building materials than blueprints, our genes are lined up, waiting to be given the order to be implemented. They are the lumber, nails, sheetrock, and fixture choices that may or may not end up being included in the physical structure. Something outside of the gene determines whether it becomes part of the building (or rebuilding) process. That command is not given at the physical level. It comes from the level of information.[15] The mechanisms that influence whether or not a gene gets used are nonphysical factors such as emotions, thoughts, and states of consciousness. Because of the Interface Effect, this is the domain of your vital body.

The true blueprint for the physical body is the vital body. It contains the energy/information instructions that determine what goes into the structure of your physical body. If you hire an architect to draw up blueprints for a new house, every detail that exists in the blueprints is eventually built into the house. The reverse is also true; everything in the structure of the finished house got there because it previously existed in the blueprints. So it is that all aspects of your physical body pre-exist in your vital body.[16] Your physical body is an exact replica of your vital body; your vital body is the "original." This Blueprint Effect of your vital body profoundly impacts your physical body—from the shape and size of your body to its ongoing health and vitality. In essence, your physical body is the stage where emotions, thoughts, and universal inergies play out. The important inergy activity is happening behind-the-scenes and your physical body is displaying the aftereffects.[17]

The Blueprint Effect helps explain why there's such a high incidence of relapse with conventional medical approaches. You can fall sick with any number of illnesses, get treated, and easily get sick again. The illness may not be truly healed because addressing only the physical counterpart potentially leaves the vital body illness intact. Although the vital body is an intelligent force with its own ways of self-correcting, it is excluded from conventional treatments. As anyone who has had cancer knows, the best that Western medicine can do is try to locate and eradicate cancer cells by removing them or destroying them, and keep doing early detection testing. We live in fear of the cancer recurring, as 22 to 55% of cancers do. Were cancer treated etherically as well, the recurrence rate could potentially be much lower. More complete healing can happen when the vital body is included in the healing process. Having a balanced and healthy vital body helps ensure a balanced and healthy physical body.

Not only is the vital body key to complete healing, it also provides an early detection system. According to the Blueprint Effect, if you have a physical ailment, it already existed in your vital body *before* it manifested on the physical level. This means you don't have to wait for an illness to show up in your physical body before you correct it. You can be pro-active by focusing on your vital body first, keeping it healthy and balanced. The next chapter explains ways to do this.

Self-Sensing Your Vital Body

The vital body is palpable on an ongoing basis to those who are finely attuned to its subtle frequency. It can be felt by anyone with a little guidance and direction. Try the following exercise to get a felt-sense of your vital body.[18] It will take about six minutes, total. It begins with your hands since they are within easy access. You are encouraged to tune in at a very subtle level. It's necessary to go very slowly and not rush the exercise. Important details can be missed if you go too fast.

Exercise: Self-Sensing Your Vital Body

- Find a quiet place in which you can focus without distraction.

- Be in a seated position, as comfortable as possible.

- Take a couple of slow, deep breaths.

- Gently close your eyes and intentionally shift your attention away from an external focus toward an internal focus, awakening your internal senses.

- Start by gently rubbing your hands together to sensitize them.

- Then, with your hands touching each other, begin *very slowly* moving your hands apart to a span ranging from 3-6 inches and as you do this, do your best to sense what is happening inside your hands and in the space between your hands. Be very attuned to the slightest sensations. Remember we are dealing with *subtle* energies. Closing your eyes can often help you self-sense better.

- Slowly and gently move your hands together and apart within a range of your hands almost touching each other to spacing them about 3-6 inches apart. Hold them close together for about 15 seconds, then slowly move them apart for about 15 seconds. Again, be very attuned to the slightest sensations.

- Then slowly move your hands further apart, beyond the 3-6 inch range, and move them back to close proximity again. Any sensations you feel will be intensified with your hands closer together and dissipate as you move your hands further apart, as you begin to lose contact with your vital body. Be keenly aware of any subtle sensations or changes.

- If you are like many people, you will be able to feel one of three things as you slowly move your hands together and apart. You might feel a change in temperature (heat or coolness); a slight resistance or force as if there were two magnets on your hands either pulling toward each other or gently pushing away; or you may feel a mild tingling, "electrical" sensation. These are the most common ways people experience the vital body. But if you experience it in another way, that's just fine. Everyone is different.

- If you're having trouble discerning any sensation, continue to move your hands further apart, out of the 3-6 inch range, and then move them back to a close proximity again to make the sensations more pronounced. If this still does not produce the desired results, it's fine. Let's try the next step.

- Now that your hands are inergetically awake, we'll begin sensing another part of your vital body, near your leg. Either leg will do. If you have a leg or knee injury, start the exercise using the uninjured leg. If both legs are injured, it doesn't matter, nor does it matter what clothing you are wearing. Because of its high frequency range, the inergy of your vital body easily passes through most clothing. Exceptions to this are discussed in the next chapter.

- Move your "sensitized" hands to the lower part of one leg, near your calf or shin.

- Place your hands about 2-3 inches from the surface of your lower leg and position your hands halfway between your ankle and knee.

- Slowly and gently move your hands close to your lower leg (about 2 inches from the surface), not touching the leg, but again, sensing the space between your hands and the surface of your leg. Hover there for about 30 seconds or more doing your best to attune to the slightest sensations. Again, closing your eyes may help.

- Then slowly move your hands slightly up and down your lower leg, slightly in and out, to get an overall sense of your etheric leg.

- Once you have a sense of the lower leg, for comparison, slowly move your hands up near your knee, again not touching your knee, but sensing into the inergy emanating from it. Hover around your knee for about 30 seconds or more, gently sensing your etheric knee.

- If you're like many people, you'll sense a difference in the inergy of your knee compared to your lower leg. Many people sense the knee as having more intense, larger, more active, or "busy" energy. If you did not experience this, it's OK.

You don't need to be an expert at sensing your vital body in order to care for it. The next chapter will guide you in health strategies for your vital body.

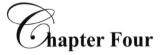

Chapter Four

Steps to a Healthy Vital Body

Many of us are trained to care for our physical bodies automatically. We get exercise, avoid fried food, shower regularly, and brush our teeth twice a day. These habits are usually so routine that we don't think much about them. Maintaining a healthy vital body can be just as easy once you are trained in habits that support vital body health. We'll learn what is helpful and harmful to the vital body so you can start making changes right away. Add to this a few exercises for the vital body and you'll have a valuable program for increased inergy. First let's find out if your vital body needs divine intervention or just a mild make-over.

Your Vital Body Health

Give yourself one point for each of the following statements you agree with.

_____ I eat microwaved food on a regular basis.

_____ My cell phone is my primary phone.

_____ Most of my clothing is made of polyester, spandex or nylon.

_____ When I'm in the sun I always use sunscreen.

_____ I regularly drink tap water.

_____ I eat a lot of canned, boxed, or other processed food.

_____ I usually don't get enough sleep.

_____ I use the popular brands of health and beauty products.

_____ I have mostly energy-saving compact fluorescent light bulbs in my home.

_____ All my shoes have plastic or synthetic soles.

_____ I drink beverages but not much water.

_____ I work under fluorescent lights.

_____ My computer is hooked up to wireless.

_____ If I'm tired I have coffee or a caffeinated drink to wake up.

Scoring Your Results

0-4 points
Your vital body has every reason to be happy with you. You are practicing good vital body hygiene and are not in the danger zone. It seems you are paying attention to the things that matter etherically and are acting accordingly. Congratulations!

5-9 points
You are borderline. Your vital body is neglected by your lifestyle choices. There is a lot you can do to help. Think about making some changes. Your vital body is depending on you to follow through.

10-14 points
Warning! You are in the danger zone. You vital body is overtaxed. If you don't intervene quickly it may become compromised. Your lifestyle choices are predisposing you to depleted inergy and potential illness. Now is the time to make some necessary changes.

There are a number of things you can do to help your vital body. Most of the tips that follow are relatively simple but can produce results in a short amount of time. Protecting your vital body from the dangers of electromagnetic pollution is the first step.

Protect Yourself From Radiation

It's hard to fathom but electromagnetic pollution increased 100 million billion times (that's 100,000,000,000,000,000) in the five-year period from 2003-2007.[1] This is not a misprint. It is a staggering number (also known as 100 quadrillion), but when you take into account the exponential increase in wireless information technologies, especially cell phones and computer networks, it becomes easier to understand. With over 2.6 billion cell phones already in use, the forecast is that consumers worldwide will continue buying mobile phones at a rate of at least a billion per year.[2] The number of text messages sent and received every day far exceeds the population of the planet. There are over 140 million active users of Facebook, a social networking website where people from all over the world gather and share profiles, stories, photos, and videos.[3] The site is growing at a rate of 230,000 registrations per day. If it were a country, Facebook would be the fourth largest in the world. Over 43 million hours are spent by users each day on that website alone. A hidden byproduct of the newly created information cosmos is the overwhelming electromagnetic pollution it produces. We are constantly being zapped. This creates particular challenges for your vital body.

Electromagnetic Radiation

Electromagnetic radiation (EMR) is a significant health concern. Many serious conditions, from cancer to Alzheimer's, are being correlated to EMR exposure. In fact, it's hard to find an illness that is not. According to biophysicist James Oschman, a world authority on energy medicine, "virtually every disease and disorder has been linked by one investigator or another to electromagnetic pollution."[4] Electric power, AM/FM, shortwave, microwave, phase modulation, terahertz technologies, WiFi, VHF, ELF, and television signals—none of these even existed 100 years ago. We are immersed in a global electronic grid. The fact is, we simply don't know what safe levels of exposure are, nor do we know the cumulative effects, or dangers of second-generation exposure. Foreshadowing what's to come, a recent study of 13,000 children shows women who use cell phones while pregnant were 54% more likely to give birth to children with behavioral problems.[5] But rather than erring on the side of caution, the issue goes almost completely unnoticed. We're part of a massive experiment in which we are the guinea pigs, along with every other living thing.

EMR is emitted by anything that uses electricity. On the physical level, EMR has been linked to brain tumors, memory loss, cardiac dysfunction, leukemia, DNA damage, immune disruption, dementia, and various forms of cancer.[6] An international consortium of 20 concerned scientists has reviewed over 2000 EMR studies and concluded that the existing standards for public safety are inadequate to protect our health. Hundreds of studies find up to a ten-fold increase in the incidence of cancer among people routinely exposed to EMR, with the most significant problems evident in long-term cell phone users. However, mainstream scientists who regard the living human body as a dead physical object argue that magnetic fields are harmless and that electric fields flow around, rather than through, the body. The harmful health effects are evident but cannot be explained by the conventional physics model. The medical community, aligned with the conventional model, comes to no conclusion and no action is taken.

Again the vital body is ignored. We are primarily energy/ information systems—not physical systems. By looking only at radiation effects on physical elements, it's as if physicists are studying a computer's hardware but missing the information software; they seem fixated on the monitor and casing but are ignoring the programming. Electromagnetic fields have profound health effects. They compromise the vital body and effectively scramble our signals, resulting in eventual physical illness. Because mainstream science does not recognize the existence of the vital body, research into EMR investigates impact on the physical body only. However, from the standpoint of the etheric (think Blueprint Effect), by the time a symptom reaches the dense physical level and manifests as an ailment, the situation is urgent.

For the vital body, less is more. Unlike the physical level, where larger inputs produce bigger responses, with the vital body smaller inputs have stronger effects.[7] In other words, you don't have to live next to a high-voltage power line or cell tower to experience significant health concerns. The inergy (energy/ information) channels that comprise the vital body are highly susceptible to damage from even low frequency fields. Oscillations of 50-60 cycles per second, the frequency range of our household power supply, have well-documented harmful effects on cellular systems.[8]

For the vital body less is more.

The good news is that EMR diminishes with distance; the bad news is that microwaves don't (this is discussed below). To help protect your vital body from EMR, it's best to keep all electrical appliances at least three feet away from your body. The electromagnetic field is one-fourth the strength at two inches out and 50 times lower at three feet.[9] Prolonged exposure is the most damaging, so be sure to move away devices you are exposed to for long periods. An electric blanket turned on all night is quite risky, with the heating coils in close proximity to your physical body, and literally enmeshed in your vital body. Even with the switch turned off the coils may emit tiny amounts of radiation. If you want to be extra safe, replace the blanket with a non-electric one and consider taking a hot bath to warm up before bed.

Pay particular attention to clearing the space around your bed. Establish an electrical-free safety zone of at least three feet in radius. Although moving a waterbed heater three feet from the waterbed is not feasible, the problem can be solved with a non-electric waterbed mattress pad designed to radiate your body's natural heat. Appliances to look out for are electronic alarm clocks, computers, televisions, portable audio players, cordless phones, and cell phones. It's best to move them, or yourself, at least three feet away. Also beware of electrical outlets near your bed, especially those close to the headboard. Reposition your bed, if possible. Consider obtaining a meter, available at nominal cost, to identify electromagnetic hotspots in your home or workplace (see Appendix B for a list of sources). With computers, place the monitor, tower, or laptop at least three feet away from you.

Cordless phones pose special problems because they use microwave frequency carrier signals (like cell phones) and interface with your head, which houses your brain. A microwave oven operates at 2450 MHz while a typical cordless phone uses 2400 MHz, a miniscule change in frequency that your vital body does not differentiate (2400 MHz means waves that vibrate 2.4 billion times per second). A cordless phone also has a radiation emitting battery pack embedded in the phone's receiver that you hold against your ear—and brain—while you're talking. Over the years, cordless phones have been manufactured for longer battery life and extended frequency ranges. All of this makes the phone's electromagnetic field more potent. For vital body health, avoid cordless phones. If you must use one, search for a model that has the lowest frequency range and limit your use of it. Better yet, don't use a cordless at all. Obtain an "old fashioned" non-electric landline telephone; the kind with a cord that you plug into a phone jack but not into an electrical socket. In case of a power outage you'll need a non-electric way to call anyway. Make this your primary phone.

If you work or live in an environment where you are exposed to daily EMR, you can help remedy the problem by getting a chip or a personal energy device (see Figure 4.1). These devices are designed to counteract electromagnetic fields (see Appendix B for a list of suppliers). Personal energy products are usually worn on the body and often take the form of a pendant placed around your neck or carried in a pocket. Chips are typically small round appliqués that adhere to the back of radiation-emitting appliances. There are also household models, about the size of a deck of cards, offering protection up to 70 feet. Some devices have been shown to reduce anxiety, improve cell tissue, and return blood cells to a healthier state, among other things.[10] There is an increased variety of protection devices available. But buyer beware: this market is new and unregulated. It is challenging to purchase a product to address invisible frequencies with effects that are subtle and subjective. When selecting what's right for you, make sure any device you purchase is backed by legitimate research and endorsed by reputable advocates.

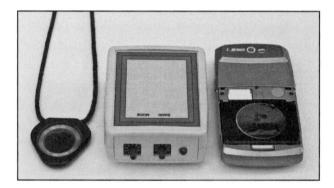

Figure 4.1 Samples of EMR protection devices including a personal energy pendant, a belt clip-on device, and a chip applique adhered to a cell phone battery pack.

Radiofrequency Radiation

So far we've addressed protecting your vital body from harmful exposure to electromagnetic frequencies. But when electricity combines with microwave frequencies, as in the case of cell phones and other wireless technologies (i.e., baby monitors, cordless phones, WiFi, PDAs, wireless computer networks, GPS, and Bluetooth), the problems are multiplied. Signal strength, frequency, and pulsed modulation combine to produce radio-frequency radiation (RFR). Wireless technologies do not operate on electricity alone. The signals that allow you to talk, view, listen, and type are transmitted on frequencies in the microwave range (300 MHz to 110 GHz).[11] These frequencies carry with them significant health concerns due to the RFR they emit.

Unlike electricity, microwaves do not diminish in short distances. They travel without wires for a considerable range and can penetrate through objects. That's why microwaved food cooks even inside containers and why your cell phone works just about anywhere, even inside buildings. The higher the frequency, the more potent the signal and the further it can travel. Microwaves are high frequency. Left uninhibited, they potentially travel infinite distances. Satellite phones and GPS (global positioning system) navigation units transmit to satellites in outer space and use microwave frequencies as their carrier signals. The only limitations on microwave frequencies are regulations that vary from country to country, with the US having some of the most lax. Standards in Europe are much stricter and the Russian standard for exposure to microwave frequencies to avoid changes in brain activity is 1000 times less than the US legal maximum.[12]

The more we use wireless technologies, the more we proliferate cell broadcast towers that are cropping up everywhere. I live on the most remote island chain on the planet (Hawaii), yet there are 23 cell towers and 62 antennas within a four-mile radius of my home.[13] A friend in San Francisco has 35 towers and 505 antennas within a two-mile radius. These are just a few of the 1.9 million cell towers/antennas that blanket the US. As wireless technology use explodes, microwaves and RFR increasingly permeate the planet. Even if you don't use wireless, your neighbors almost certainly do and that exposes you to RFR. Schools, airports, office complexes, hotels, hospitals, and entire cities are going wireless. When the vital body is constantly compromised, physical malady is bound to follow. This affects humans, wildlife, and plant life as well because living plants and animals also have a vital body.

RFR from cell phones has special impact when you use your phone inside a car or other enclosed metal space. The dangers of putting metal in a microwave oven are well known. If you've made this mistake you probably remember what happens. The sparks fly because microwaves cannot travel through metal. When you use your cell phone inside a car, the phone transmits microwave frequencies inside the car. The car, being metal on all sides, traps some of the microwaves, potentially turning your car into a mobile microwave oven with you inside it.[14] Because the car is moving, the phone surges in power as it repeatedly searches for new relay antennas. Using a phone with an external antenna port and installing an antenna on the outside of your car could help (see Appendix B for supplier).

In June of 2008 four videos appeared on YouTube that showed a group of friends allegedly popping kernels of popcorn with their cell phones. In less than a week, the videos were viewed more than a million times around the world and spurred copycat experiments with people trying to replicate the effect using more phones or other kinds of foods, like eggs. They were unsuccessful. The original videos turned out to be a viral marketing campaign put forth by the BlueTooth group, a wireless alternative typically used in clip-on ear headsets, apparently fueling fears about conventional cell phone hazards.

Although wireless clip-on ear devices appear to emit less EMR than cell phones, they are not recommended because of RFR hazards. They are clipped onto your ear (next to your brain), usually for long periods (RFR is cumulative), and contain a receiver, a transmitter, and operate within microwave frequency ranges that can interrupt the information processing capacity of cellular functioning.[15] Hands-free headsets that are required in a growing number of states for cell phone use while driving are also potentially harmful. The copper wiring in some headsets acts as an antenna, increasing the radiation and directing it straight into your head.

If you must use a cell phone, there are important guidelines to follow to protect your vital body. Below are natural and barrier methods for, tongue-in-cheek, "safe cell" practices. Combine both methods for maximum protection. Some suppliers of the products listed can be found in Appendix B.

Natural Methods for Safe Cell:[16]

- **The cell is not for kids.** No matter what advertisers may say, do not allow children to use a cell phone, except for emergencies. Not only are children more susceptible to RFR, the health effects of long-term, cumulative use are of particular concern. Do not put a wireless baby monitor near your child's bed and don't use a cell phone if you are pregnant.

- **Limit cell use.** Don't use the cell phone for more than a few minutes at a time. Turn it on only to establish contact, then turn it off. Use a landline with a corded phone for longer conversations.

- **Keep the cell off your body.** Don't keep your cell phone in your pocket, in your bra, on your belt or in your bed. Keep it as far away from your body as possible and transport it in a bag or briefcase.

- **Use speaker-mode.** If you can't use the speaker-mode, wait until your party has picked up before putting the phone to your ear. Switch ears regularly to spread out your exposure.

- **Text message instead of call.** This keeps the phone away from your body mass. Put the phone down after sending as it emits radiation/signals even when texting.

- **Avoid other's cells.** Keep a safe distance from other people's cell phones and avoid using yours in places where you expose others to second-hand radiation/signals.

- **No cell in the car.** Don't use a cell phone inside a car or other enclosed metal space due to the microwave effect described above.

- **Keep the cell off** (or in off-line mode) until you need to use it. Make calls and access all your voicemails, emails and texts at once and turn it off again.

- **Use a safe cell position.** If you must carry a cell phone on you and cannot use a barrier method (see below), position the phone so the keypad is facing toward your body and the back of the phone is facing outward. This may help the frequencies to flow away from, rather than through, your body.

- **Beware of movement.** Don't use a cell phone when moving at high speed (i.e., in a car or subway). This will cause it to ramp up in power as it repeatedly searches for new relay towers.

- **Beware of a weak signal.** Don't use a cell phone when the signal is weak as this will cause it to ramp up power in an attempt to establish a clearer connection.

- **Beware of SAR.** Don't mistake a low SAR (Specific Absorption Rate) rating for cell phone safety. The FCC and mainstream science do not recognize the existence of the vital body, thus, SAR ratings are meaningless in terms of inergy health.

Barrier Methods for Safe Cell:[17]

- **Use a frequency exposure shield** to block and deflect frequencies away from your body. These low-cost belt and pocket shields are made of a thin, laminated screen fabric. You can even buy the fabric and cut out your own design. Of course, you cannot cover your entire phone with it or the phone won't work.

- **Use a hollow-tube headset.** By interrupting the ambient flow, hollow tube headsets can significantly cut radiation compared to wired headsets.

- **Use a wire protection guard** with your headset, even with a hollow tube unit. This small ferrite bead clamps on to the wire and helps prevent your headset from becoming an antenna that increases radiation when it touches your body.

- **Use ear-bud shields.** If you cannot use a hollow tube headset, using ear-bud shields on your wired headset can cut the flow of frequencies into your head.

- **Install a car antenna** and use an antenna-compatible cell phone if you must use your phone in the car.

Remember, practicing these methods does not mean your cell is safe. Abstinence is the best protection.

Be In Natural Light

In addition to EMR and RFR, your vital body is particularly sensitive to another form of energy, namely, light. The vital body needs natural sunlight. The sun produces a certain type of nutrient-rich inergy this body thrives on. Winter depression, or Seasonal Affective Disorder (SAD), and the lack of vitamin D evident in people who do not get enough natural sunlight are just the tip of the iceberg. Lack of sun has been linked to everything from organ cancers, flues, cardiovascular disease, and infections to premature aging, mental decline, memory loss, impaired brain functioning and autism.[18] The recent UV scare that has people covering their bodies and slathering their skin has led to an anemic vital body. While I am not advocating tossing out the sunscreen and wearing only your birthday suit to the beach, it is important for the vital body to get some natural light. The equivalent of ten minutes of afternoon sunlight on your skin every day is recommended.

Whether it's sun-phobia or busy lifestyle, more people are staying indoors and for longer periods. Instead of exposure to natural sunlight, the vital body is fed an artificial diet. Artificial light is substandard and often lacking in many of the essential nutrients of the sun. Through use of a spectroscope it's possible to analyze the ingredients of various light sources. Natural sunlight contains all the colors of the spectrum in uniform frequency patterns.

Fluorescent light, however, contains drastically inconsistent frequencies such as large energy peaks in the yellow, green and violet ranges; it also emits more electromagnetic radiation than incandescent light.[19] This is of special concern because florescent tube lighting is so prevalent in public places and compact fluorescent bulbs are increasingly used for home lighting. In electrician's parlance, inconsistent energy frequencies are commonly referred to as *dirty energy*. Through continuous exposure to fluorescent lighting, the vital body is fed the inergy-equivalent of contaminated food.

It's tempting to remedy the problem by using modified light bulbs that are marketed and labeled "full-spectrum." Sadly, even so-called full-spectrum lighting is bereft.[20] These bulbs produce light that is virtually lacking in yellow frequencies, an essential nutrient for the vital body. The same is true for full-spectrum fluorescents. They are lacking in yellow as well as red, plus they produce dirty energy. In other words, they are both nutritionally deficient and contaminated. Often these factors are hidden in advertising when manufacturers' color charts depict "averaged" frequency levels that mask the discrepancies. Energy efficient warm-white LED bulbs show promise as being closer to full-spectrum.

Next to the sun, the healthiest lighting is the common household incandescent light bulb because it comes closest to replicating the balanced frequency spectrum of natural sunlight.[21] This seems a simple solution to the lighting problem. However, some states and even entire countries are in the process of prohibiting use of these bulbs. California and Canada are considering legislation to phase out the sale of incandescent bulbs by 2012 and Australia's goal is 2010. The European Union is considering a similar plan. Requiring everyone to replace incandescent light bulbs with fluorescents is prompted by energy conservation concerns. But this may be harmful, not only for inergy health, it's potentially bad for the environment too. Many fluorescent light bulbs contain toxic mercury, which could end up in the environment unless extensive recycling efforts are mandated to accompany these changes. Hopefully this will happen.

Just as good food is good medicine, good light is the vital body's medicine. Natural sunlight contains a rainbow of colors. Each color has specific properties and therapeutic effects.[22] This is especially true for light received through the eyes. It's best to expose your eyes to natural daylight as much as possible. Again, sensibility must be used, as I am not advocating damaging your eyes by over-exposure to harsh sunlight or glare. But many people habitually wear sunglasses to the extent that natural sunlight rarely reaches their eyes. Instead, the colored light of the sunglass lens acts as an etherically altering substance, the inergy-equivalent of constantly medicating your vital body. If you must wear sunglasses, choose a neutral shade, such as gray, to minimize this effect.

Eat Vitalized Food

Food manufacturers these days are fond of using the word *energy* to market their products. We have energy drinks, energy blends and bars with power. The fact is most manufactured food is dead. Just as the human body has a vital interface, so do the bodies of living plants and animals. This carries over into the food you eat. As important as the nutritional content of the food is its inergy content. If you want the most inergy mileage out of your food, it's best to eat foods that are flowing with vitality and life-force. A general rule of thumb: the closer to the earth, the more vitality. This means eating lots of fresh fruits and vegetables and avoiding four inergy thieves: processing, chemicalizing, microwaving, and modifying.

Foods that are heavily processed are inergetically dead. They are far removed from their life source, the earth, and therefore lack inergetic content. What we find on our grocery store shelves are products of the food science industry, most of which have proven to be less beneficial—and sometimes even harmful—to health.[23] Here is a short list of some common processed food ingredients to avoid:[24]

- **Sodium nitrite**: A chemical that helps artificial coloring hold its color. It's been linked to cancer and is found in processed meats like hot dogs, bacon, and sausage.

- **Hydrogenated oils**: Sometimes called "plastic fat," they make oils last longer to extend product shelf life. They are converted to trans fat in the body.

Hydrogenated oils have been linked to heart disease, nutritional deficiencies, and the deterioration of cells. They are found in a vast array of processed foods including cookies, crackers, chips, cereals, and margarine.

- **Aspartame, monosodium glutamate, and yeast extract**: These were the original names of these artificial flavor enhancers but when consumers caught on and began to avoid them they were re-labeled with new names, such as autolyzed vegetable protein, hydrolyzed vegetable protein, calcium caseinate, sodium caseinate, and textured protein. Called *excitotoxins,* these substances are linked to nerve damage and autoimmune disorders. They are found in diet sodas, soups, salad dressings, processed meats and processed vegetarian foods.

Some laboratory engineered foods contain no harmful ingredients at all. Instead, they are formulated and infused with all the vitamins and nutrients thought necessary to sustain life. But in the absence of life-force, which can only come from living things, these "techno-foods" are inergetically empty. Eating for the physical body alone does not work. Since we are primarily comprised of inergy, feeding the vital body with inergy rich foods is of utmost importance.

Our food supply is being deadened on multiple levels. The dangers of commercially grown foods, with chemical pesticides and herbicides, are well known. Chemical food additives and preservatives represent an additional level of life-force removal. Hormone and pharmaceutically medicated animals add yet another layer to the problem. Then there is irradiation. From the standpoint of inergy, however, genetic alteration is perhaps the most problematic.

Many of us are consuming genetically modified (GMO) food without even knowing it. Already in the US food supply, 89% of soybeans, 75% of canola, and 61% of corn are genetically modified.[25] When you consider how many products contain corn (corn oil, corn starch, corn syrup, high fructose corn syrup, and corn syrup solids) or soybeans (soy lecithin, soybean oil, soy protein, and tofu), the scope of the situation is daunting. The FDA has even considered allowing both milk and meat from cloned animals to be on the market *without labeling it as such.* Altering food at the level of genetics means altering the information content of the food. The plant is no longer "programmed" to be itself. Instead, modified genetic codes are created, ones that merge plant life with pesticides or plastics and do not derive from the innate intelligence of living nature. They are based on the limited knowledge of the food science industry, and often motivated by corporate interests. To use Einstein's famous quote, "God does not play dice." But humans do. We are gambling with our own lives and the lives of other living things.

Inergy-depleted foods undernourish your vital body in two ways. First, they deprive it of essential inergy by not supplying it in the first place. Second, they can act to steal inergy from your vital body. Fabricating foods—altering them through combinations of genetic mutation, canning, freezing, fortifying, chemicalizing, dehydrating, preserving, storing—depletes their inergy content. Each process removes some of the vital life-force from the food.

Hungry foods can rob your inergy.

This leaves the food hungry, so to speak. Being inergy deprived, the hungry food can rob inergy from your vital body to compensate for its own deficiency. This may explain why you can feel de-energized right after eating. A similar effect occurs with microwaved food, as the microwaves directly alter the inergy content of the food.

If you are consuming foods that are low in inergy your vital body is not satisfied. This can evoke a feeling of craving so you go after more food, not realizing what the craving is truly about. The vital body wants inergy not calories: inergy comes from inergy. The craving does not go away, so you feel compelled to eat more. At the same time, having a small amount of food that is high in inergy can evoke a sense of fullness without having to consume a lot of it. Eating high inergy foods can be quite satisfying on one condition: focus your attention primarily on the inergy content and not on the physical components. In other words, train yourself to "think inergy" when it comes to food.

Most of us approach what we eat on a purely physical level. Either we're seeing food in terms of calories or fat, or in terms of our external senses—how the food looks, tastes and smells. But artificial ingredients, food dyes, and flavor enhancers make food products deceiving. You can no longer trust your external senses. Focusing exclusively on the physical level leaves us victim to the ever-changing fads of the food science industry and to the clutches of clever advertisers adept at altering products to appeal to the external senses. Weight problems can easily develop if we get caught up in the physical aspects of food and neglect the inergy aspects.

If you train yourself to think in terms of inergy, you approach food primarily with your internal senses. Use self-sensing to discern when you're hungry and what you're hungry for. Use your intent to focus on the inergy content of what's available. Self-sense your entire system's responses to certain foods. Instead of counting calories and agonizing about cholesterol, you can have fun with food and bring joy (a high frequency inergy) to your eating experience. Experiment with the inergy sensing exercise from the previous chapter (in which you activated your etheric hands) and try it on different foods. Practice becoming attuned to the inergy frequencies of various foods and let the physical aspects drop to the background. This simple shift in perception—from the physical to the inergetic—can mean the difference between having a fit, vitalized physical body and a sluggish, overweight or weak, depleted one.

Save Your Skin

If you put something on your skin it stays outside of your body because your skin is external, right? We've all seen the label:

For External Use Only, which means you can put it on your skin but you shouldn't eat it. Inergetically speaking, though, *on* means *in*. Your vital body does not end at your skin; it extends beyond your physical body for two to three inches, creating an energy/information field around you. Your vital body communicates with the external environment via your skin cells. Rather than being a barrier, your skin is more like a sponge. What you put on your skin or within several inches of it is immediately registered by your vital body and its "information-sensors," your cells.

Body cells do not function as we have been taught. Cell behavior is not determined by the cell nucleus, what was once understood to be the brain of the cell. Instead, we now know that cells are information-based transducers; they form an excitable medium, much like the liquid crystals that comprise an interactive computer screen.[26] They take information from their environment and translate those messages into biochemical signals and other elements of the language of biology. Through receptor sites on the cell membrane, cells act as tiny computer chips that are programmed by factors *outside* the cell. The lines of distinction between internal and external simply do not exist, right down to the cellular level.

This seamlessness was first documented in skin cells and extends all the way to the level of genetics.[27] Our biological functioning and gene activity are intrinsically linked to information from the environment that gets downloaded into the cell. With skin cells, the information input from the immediate environment involves what you put on or near your skin. Your vital body registers the inergy content of the substance and is affected before the substance even touches your skin. Your skin cells amplify the energy/information and translate it directly into your physical body at the level of cellular behavior.

Since we are primarily energy/information systems, we are prone to the problem of mixed messages. It used to be that chemicals were isolated to industrial use and household products were pure, made of natural food-based substances. The lines between the two were clear and distinct. Your vital body knew if it was being exposed to a toxin or a friendly substance. Now that chemical companies have taken over most "health and beauty" products (and food and clothing as well) chemicals have found their way into just about everything.

Most soaps, lotions, sunscreens, toothpastes, shave creams, shampoos, first-aid creams, and cosmetics are manufactured by chemical companies and contain a mixture of sweet smelling, skin soothing ingredients that are laced with toxic chemicals.[28] When you apply them on your skin, your vital body immediately registers the information and gets a double message: the product is simultaneously alluring and harmful. It's the proverbial wolf in sheep's clothing, the Trojan horse. Because of the mixed message, your vital body is tricked into letting toxins straight into your system.

It's not good to let strangers into your body. Avoid anything with names you don't recognize as safe. Get in the habit of reading ingredient labels for everything you put on your skin or breathe in. Hair products (coloring, hairspray, perms) and nail products (nail polish and polish remover) are especially harsh. If your work requires that you expose yourself to known toxins on a regular basis wear protective clothing/gloves and remember to protect your lungs too. Even from a purely physical standpoint, your skin is a semi-permeable membrane (like your tongue). Whatever touches your skin goes directly into your system. Whether it's industrial strength cleansers, automotive oil, dish soap, household glue, or hand sanitizer—you might as well be eating it. The bottom line is, if you wouldn't put it in your mouth, don't put it on your skin.

Wear Healthy Fabrics

Some clothing is inergetically healthy and some isn't. The determining factor is the extent to which the fabric blocks or allows inergy flow. Your vital body receives and assimilates inergy from the environment via the seven major inergy centers and is dependent on that inergy to function. If the vital body is covered with inergy-blocking clothing it cannot breathe, so to speak. This taxes it and can lead to a devitalized state. In general, natural fibers allow inergy to flow. Fabrics that are plant and animal derived allow inergy to travel through them without blocking it because, like humans, living plants and animals are inergy based (they also have a vital body).

Inergy-Friendly Fabrics
    Cotton
    Wool
    Hemp
    Cashmere
    Ramie
    Silk
    Linen
    Rayon/Modal
    Bamboo

Cotton is still on the inergy-friendly list but this may be changing soon, as 83% of cotton is now genetically modified.[29] There could come a point in the future where the genetic code of cotton will be altered to the extent that it no longer resembles cotton enough to sustain inergy health. Rayon is a special case because it is not a synthetic or a natural fiber. It is an artificial fabric manufactured from natural fibers (mostly plant-derived cellulose), making most rayon inergy friendly. This includes modal, which is in the rayon family.

Fabrics that block inergy are chemically derived synthetics. The inergy-blocker list is ever increasing as the materials science industry is constantly coming up with new formulas and new names. The chemical companies that manufacture and sell the synthetic fabrics heavily fund research into new synthetics. Be on the lookout for trademarked fabric names (which are not included on this list) as a trademark indicates the fabric is synthetic, not natural.

Inergy-Blocking Fabrics
    Nylon

Microfiber
Polyester
Acrylic
Spandex
Acetate
Olefin
Modacrylic

Because of the many inergy channels flowing in your feet, inergy-blocking shoes should also be avoided. Choose shoes with natural soles made of rubber or cork and avoid shoes that are plastic or synthetic. Better yet, go shoeless sometimes. Fifteen minutes of barefoot contact with a grassy or other natural area upon arrival to your new location is said to counteract the effects of jet lag.[30]

Drink Live Water

On planet Velara III a terraforming station discovers a microscopic life form within the sand of the planet. The silica-based creature kills one of the colonists to save itself from being destroyed. The crew of the Starship *Enterprise* utilize their universal translator apparatus to communicate and hear the silica creature refer to humans as "ugly bags of mostly water."[31] Although the assessment of ugliness may be debatable, the fact that we are mostly water is not. The physical body is about 80% water. Your brain is the most water-consuming organ in your body; the next largest consumer is the lung.[32]

Water is a special substance that has unique properties. There is nothing else like it on the planet. In the human body, the importance of water cannot be overemphasized. Water has a dual effect in that it both conditions and is conditioned by the cells and tissues, facilitating information to travel at light-speed within your body.[33] Water is an essential medium through which inergy flows throughout your system. As such, it is intrinsic to inergy health. However, not just any water. Pure, fresh, vitalized water is best.

Water has the capacity to take on the inergy imprint of what it comes in contact with. This is most evident in the field of homeopathy where water is routinely imprinted with the "inergy-signature" of substances that are successfully used in healing a variety of illnesses.[34] Structured water devices employ the same principle (see Appendix C). In addition to adapting to substances, water is also highly susceptible to words and human intent. Perhaps this is why religious people have been making and using holy water since time immemorial. The research of Masaru Emoto and others verifies the capacity of water to change its structure in response to concentrated thoughts and words.[35] Using high-speed photography Dr. Emoto showed that crystals formed in frozen water take on specific shapes when exposed to certain information.

By the time it reaches your household tap, most water has passed through someone's sewer or a toxic industrial conduit.[36] Water is endlessly recycled in cities, and chlorine, a known hazard even to inanimate objects, is routinely added. Bottled water is unregulated so you don't know for sure what you are drinking, and the leeching effect of plastic from the bottle into the water makes it doubly undesirable. In addition, most bottled water sits in dark warehouses for long periods and eventually ends up bathed in fluorescent lights on store shelves. Chemicalizing water, trapping it in plastic bottles for prolonged periods, storing it in darkness or artificial light, all these factors combine to effectively kill the water. Dead water is unable to fully perform its function as an inergy conductor.

The solution is not an easy one. For inergy health, the best water is clean, moving, exposed to natural sunlight, and has just emerged from the earth on its own. This type of water has high frequency inergy vibration and is teeming with vitality. I am describing natural spring water, of course, but not many of us can hike out and gather pristine spring-fed water to quench our thirst. Increased demand and expanding urban sprawl make water that meets this description scarce.

You can take control of your water by using a home water system. This way you know what you're getting in terms of purity and need not rely on the claims of an unregulated bottled water industry. You'll also avoid the proliferation of plastic bottles. Check specifications before buying a filtration unit to make sure the filter removes a long list of known toxins and not just superficial impurities (see Appendix C for water technology suppliers). Consider getting a filter for the shower too as your skin is a great absorber. Look for research to back up claims. In general, you get what you pay for. Pour-through pitcher type filters do only a surface cleaning of the water. Under-the-counter models have more filter capacity and clean better. Reverse osmosis units work well for cleaning the water but, like distillation methods, they also remove essential minerals that the body needs and so are not recommended.

In addition to filtration, ionization units that restructure the water are anti-oxidizing and allow you to adjust the pH of the water. This is important because alkalinizing your body through water and food choices appears to have significant health benefits. Although a full discussion is beyond the scope of this chapter, it is worth mentioning that the Japanese Ministry of Health recognizes ionized alkaline water as a medical treatment and has approved certain ionization units as medical devices.

Recharge with Sleep

Lack of sleep has become a national health crisis. Recent studies link sleep deprivation to heart disease, cancer, diabetes, obesity, fatal accidents and moodiness.[37] In fact, evidence is that lack of sleep disrupts *every* physiologic function. People who routinely get less than six hours of sleep per night die younger. Emotional functioning is also impaired by reduced sleep.[38] With nearly half of all Americans reporting difficulty sleeping on a regular basis, the problem has reached epidemic proportions. However, sleep is a mystery that modern medicine is at a loss to resolve. Researchers can find nothing in the physical body that would require it to sleep.

However, when the vital body is brought into the picture, again the mystery is solved. Sleep is primarily an inergy activity. During sleep the physical body rests but the vital body is working. It's busy repairing and rebuilding the dense physical body while the emotional and mental bodies are restored through dreaming.[39] Experiences during the day create a kind of friction between your physical body with its low frequency substance and your higher frequency bodies—the vital, emotional, mental and universal. That inergetic friction translates as fatigue and is best remedied through sleep. Although it may sound paradoxical: if you want more inergy, sleep.

In our over-stimulated lives, unfortunately, sleep does not come easily. One in every four Americans takes some kind of sleep aid. Evidence is that long-term use of sleep aids can make the body dependent and it may lose its ability to sleep without them.[40] Just as artificial food and clothing are detrimental to the vital body, so is artificially induced sleep. During natural sleep, your vital body is actively repairing your physical body and processing inergies from your other bodies. Sleep medications force sleep by shutting down the physical body but this may prevent the vital body from doing its important restoration work. Artificial sleep aids may also interrupt the natural dream cycle in which the emotional body figures prominently.

Because the vital body interfaces with the other bodies, sleep restores us on all levels. Instead of pushing through a dip in inergy, try taking a short nap. Minor physical ailments (a sniffle, a headache, a scratchy throat) can often be repaired through sleep. Countries in which afternoon siestas are common are shown to have a lower incidence of heart disease.[41] Companies are getting the hint and adding nap rooms to corporate offices. If you are one of the unfortunates who cannot sleep, try the Inergy Pretzel exercise described in the next section (Vital Body Exercises). The inability to sleep can often be remedied by correcting an over-inergy flow in the vital body.

To summarize, here is a list of what you can do to help your vital body.

What to Do
Protect Yourself From Radiation
Be In Natural Light
Eat Vitalized Food
Save Your Skin
Wear Healthy Fabrics
Drink Live Water
Recharge with Sleep
Exercise Your Vital Body (see below)

Vital Body Exercises

Just as your physical body needs exercise to stay fit and healthy, so does your vital body. In addition to following the guidelines above, the exercises that follow can help tune-up your vital body. When you first go to the gym, you may find that you are out of shape and can't do much. But if you stay with a fitness program, you can strengthen your body and increase stamina. It's important to stay with any exercise routine for your system to incorporate the changes. By practicing the following exercises on a regular basis, you can train your vital body to be strong and resilient, better able to withstand inergy disturbances. Daily practice of each exercise is recommended. You can complete the entire routine in about seven minutes per day, total.

Inergy Shower

There's nothing like a shower to refresh and recharge. This exercise invites you to start your day with an inergy shower as well, to help cleanse and invigorate your vital body. While you are in the regular shower, standing under the water, use your intent to tune-in to your vital body and visualize the shower recharging you.

Exercise: Inergy Shower
Application: For use while showering
Time: 1-2 minutes

- Close your eyes and use your intent to tune in to your vital body. Then visualize and feel the water as an inergy shower. Sense and see the shower-spray as streams of radiant inergy to vitalize and recharge you. Allow the vibrant streams to pour over your body, feel the inergy as it cleanses your vital body.

- Spend at least 1-2 minutes in the inergy shower, bathing in its glowing beams.

Inergy Breath

This exercise[42] works as a quick pick-up for those times when your inergy dips during the day. It can be done discretely just about anywhere and takes only a few minutes. The exercise is best done in a seated position with both feet on the floor.

Exercise: Inergy Breath
Application: Daily and when needed to revitalize
Time: 5 minutes

- Close your eyes and relax your physical body.

- Take a couple of slow, deep breaths.

- Focus all your attention on your breath, so you can feel yourself breathing from the inside out.

- Then shift your attention to your left foot.

- Visualize that your left foot is bathing in a small pool of inergy. Do your best to sense and see the inergy.

- On the next inhalation breathe the inergy up through the bottom of your left foot, up your left leg, up the left side of your body, and out through the top of your left-brain hemisphere.

- Repeat this breathing of the inergy several times on the left side.

- Pause and notice any difference you now feel between the left and right sides of your body. Any difference you experience is due to the power of your intent and your vital body's response to that.

- Then shift to breathing the inergy on the right side and repeat the sequence above several times on your right side, starting with your right foot.

- Optional: Breathe the inergy up one side of your body and then cross-over and breathe it down the other side, then back up, repeating this several times.

Inergy Pretzel

When inergy is out of balance we can feel devitalized and tired. However, it's possible at times to feel over-energized, frazzled or "wired" instead. This can be most troubling if it occurs at bedtime. The following exercise[43] has been known to help by balancing an over-inergy flow. Crossing the arms and legs in the pretzel-like manner described connects the major power lines that run through the hands and legs, helping to redistribute and equalize the inergy.[44] The technique is best done in a seated position but can also be done lying down (that is, in bed if you are trying to fall asleep).

Exercise: Inergy Pretzel
Application: Daily for general toning, and as needed to
help with relaxation or sleep
Time: 2-3 minutes

- Breathe gently and deeply throughout the exercise.

- Touch your tongue to the roof of your mouth behind
  your front teeth.

- Cross your legs at the ankles. It doesn't matter which
  leg is on top.

Step 1

- Stretch your arms out in front of you with your hands
  back to back touching each other and your palms
  facing outward. Drop one hand slightly (doesn't
  matter which hand), cross your arms, and move your
  palms toward each, clasping your hands together.
  Rotate your clasped hands down and inward, toward
  your chest, and rest them there (see Figure 4.2).

- Hold this for about 1 minute, then release your arms
  and uncross your legs.

Step 2

- Gently touch the tips of your fingers and thumbs
  together (see Figure 4.3); keep both feet firmly on the
  floor. Keep your tongue on the roof of your mouth.

- Hold this for about 1 minute.

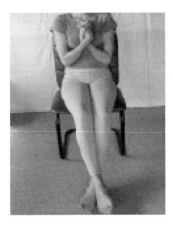

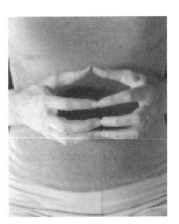

Inergy Pretzel

Figure 4.2 (Left)
The arm and
leg positions for
Step 1

Figure 4.3
(Right) The
hand position
for Step 2

Collar, Lips and Tail

The energy/information channels in your vital body are susceptible to signal scrambling from a variety of sources (i.e., elements from the environment such as those described above as well as emotions and thoughts). When this happens, foggy thinking and fatigue can result. This exercise[45] helps promote clear communication in the vital/physical interface.

Rub the points indicated in Figures 4.4, 4.5 and 4.6 near the collarbone, lips, and tailbone with medium pressure. Since the exercise works with active inergies that move about and are responsive, it's not necessary to locate the physical points exactly, as long as you are within about two inches.

Exercise: Collar + Lips + Tail
Application: Daily for general toning, and as needed to help with foggy thinking or fatigue
Time: 2 minutes

- Breathe gently and deeply throughout the exercise.

- **Step 1**: Place one hand on your abdomen with your palm centered over your navel. It doesn't matter which hand you start with.

- Use your other hand to locate the "knobs" on either side of your breastbone just below your collarbone (see Figure 4.4).[46] These knobs feel like little indentations just under your collarbone on the outside edge of your sternal notch.

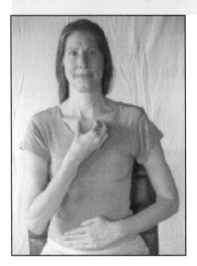

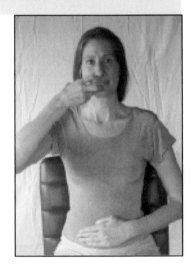

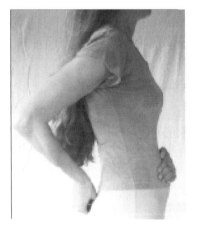

Figure 4.4 (Upper left)
Step 1: Rub the "knobs" on either side of the collarbone.

Figure 4.5 (Upper right)
Step 2: Rub the points above the upper lip and below the lower lip.

Figure 4.6 (Lower left)
Step 3: Rub just above the tailbone.

- Rub both knobs for about 15-30 seconds. Then switch hands and repeat the rubbing.

- **Step 2**: Keep one hand on your navel and move your other hand to your mouth area. Center your index finger above your upper lip and your middle finger below your lower lip (see Figure 4.5). You may use different fingers if you wish; just make sure to stimulate the lip points.[47]

- Rub the two points for about 15-30 seconds. Then switch hands and repeat the rubbing.

- **Step 3**: The final step is to keep one hand on your navel and move your other hand to the back of your body to your tailbone area. Locate the flat area in the center just above your tailbone (see Figure 4.6).[48]

- Rub the tailbone area for about 15-30 seconds. Then switch hands and repeat the rubbing.

If you want to revitalize your inergy and are in a situation where you're unable to do the exercises, try this simple shift in perception. Remind yourself of your vital body and your primary nature as non-physical. Use your intent to tap in to your inergy source. Visualize yourself as an inergy being, comprised of extreme high frequency inergies vibrating freely and easily. Use self-sensing to bring your attention to your inergy nature. Remember what you are. If you are like most people, you will find that shifting your perception to that of inergy allows you to instantly feel lighter. This experience is available to you whenever you choose.

Just as your physical body responds to exercise, so will your vital body. By practicing these exercises and adopting the habits outlined, you can help your vital body to be robust and fit. This contributes to overall health and wellbeing because your vital body is the gateway to your other bodies. Now that you have a sense of your vitality, let's look at your emotional body in the next chapter to discover its role in your inergy health.

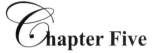

Chapter Five

Your Emotional Body

Rachel was conceived during a one-night stand between two people who barely knew each other. They married several months before she was born and proceeded to fight on a regular basis throughout her childhood. They would yell at each other, throw things, and eventually one parent would storm off for several days only to return and repeat the pattern. Rachel and her younger brother would try to wedge themselves in between their parents to stop the fights. Over the years they had some success in diffusing the chaos by yelling back and threatening to call the police, but they were never able to bring harmony to their family.

     Rachel is currently in a long-term relationship with Ryan. Ryan grew up in a similar situation with his parents continuously at each other's throats. His father's rage was so intense that young Ryan was no match for it. He learned to cope by retreating to his room and absorbing himself in books.

     Now when Rachel and Ryan have disagreements, he under-reacts by going silent and ignoring her in favor of his computer. She over-reacts by yelling and blaming. When Ryan is unresponsive, it taps in to Rachel's fear of being left, which causes her to flare up even more. Despite her small stature, she lashes out in a big way. This triggers Ryan's fear of anger and attack. He decides things are too heated and flatly tells her to calm down and relax. She screams at him to have a heart. Eventually he just leaves, playing out her worst fear. He returns hours later to remain sullen and silent, his large frame once again hunched over his computer.

Despite coming from similar backgrounds, Ryan and Rachel react quite differently to stress in their relationship. These differences can be understood in terms of their distinct personalities and coping mechanisms developed through their growing up experiences. However, if we go deeper to discover the inergy (energy/information) influences behind their behaviors, we encounter the emotional body.

The emotional body occupies the frequency band in between the vital/physical and mental bodies. This body is one of the most active, yet most misunderstood. It links us to the physical world as well as to our inner being. It allows us to sense desires and emotions (i.e., pleasant or unpleasant) and plays a role in intuition. It is also responsible for a vast array of physical ailments, as it possesses inergies so powerful they do not easily diminish over time. In studies sponsored by the Centers for Disease Control involving thousands of adults, emotionally stressful childhood experiences have been linked to the leading causes of death 50 years later.[1] This points to the powerful effect of the emotional body on the physical and the importance of properly caring for this complex body.

Universal Body

Mental Body

Emotional Body

Vital/Physical Body

The interrelationship among the bodies is a two-way process. The emotional body influences the physical and mental bodies as well as being influenced by them. An emotional upset can easily get translated into physical pain or illness. You may become nervous and end up with a stomachache, or experience frustration and then get a headache. An activated emotional body can also contaminate your thought process, producing distorted ideas and faulty reasoning. In turn, the emotional body is highly influenced by its neighboring bodies. When you are in physical pain, it's easy to become emotional. You may feel happy at the start of your day but if the lower back flares up or a throbbing headache sets in, the happiness can quickly dissolve into irritability. Similarly, if you are in a bad mood and go to the gym for a good physical workout, you tend to feel brighter.

Because of its proximity to the mental level, the emotional body is also influenced by thoughts. If you think stressful thoughts, your emotional body begins to vibrate at a similar frequency and corresponding feelings get evoked. Once that happens your emotional body can, in turn, influence your mental body. Stressful thoughts get reinforced, creating a self-perpetuating loop of stressful thinking and feeling.

Amplifier Loops

The concept of resonance is important to understanding the overall functioning of your inergy (energy/information) bodies. Resonance is a physics term referring to the amplification that occurs between two equal frequencies, as happens with sound. Let's say I have a tuning fork that is calibrated to the key of D. I strike the tuning fork and it begins to emanate the D tone. At that moment you happen to walk into the room holding a fork that is also tuned to D. Without you doing anything, your fork will begin to vibrate on its own, emitting the D tone as well, because it is resonant with my fork; it is calibrated to the same frequency. If you are holding a fork that is tuned to any other frequency, nothing will happen because there is no resonance.

When your mental body produces stressful thoughts, those thoughts vibrate at a specific frequency. Each thought carries a particular "inergetic tone." If your emotional body has any parallel frequencies, which it usually does, it will begin to vibrate in harmony and stressful feelings get activated. Your mental and emotional bodies become resonant, much like the two tuning forks. Once that happens, the stressful emotions reinforce similar thoughts. An amplification loop is created in which the mental and emotional bodies feed off each other, forming a self-perpetuating resonance pattern. Left uninterrupted, these patterns can cause you to spiral to extremes, such as depression or hostility. Similar amplifier effects can also occur between people. In the next chapter we will discuss ways to interrupt these loops.

Just as your physical body has its own unique shape and dimensions so does your emotional body. Like the physical body, emotional bodies are prone to weight problems and to being out of shape. However, there's no correlation between the size of your physical and emotional bodies. You can have a petite physical body yet an obese emotional body, and vice versa, or they may be similar in size.

The emotional body plays a major role in romance. Within a relational context, the emotional body becomes highlighted and any size difference between two bodies is enhanced, as intimate relationships are based on feelings—feelings of attraction. Although the emotional body is capable of myriad feelings, essentially all of its domain can be condensed down to two primary inergy forces— attraction and repulsion. We are inergetically attracted to things we desire and pushed away (repulsed) by those we don't. Since what we desire can change in an instant, the emotional body is prone to turbulence and agitation.

Feelings Are Food

Similar to your physical body, the size, shape, weight and overall condition of your emotional body are largely determined by what you feed it. Metaphorically speaking, feelings are food for this body. Stressful feelings are heavy because they vibrate slowly, at low frequency ranges, toward the material-substance end of the inergy continuum. They are like rich, fat-saturated food, inergetically dense, causing excess weight in the emotional body. Pleasant feelings are light, yet dynamic. They are like super-foods, rich in phyto-nutrients, teaming with vitality, nourishment and life.

Renowned psychiatrist David Hawkins, M.D., Ph.D., has logged the frequencies of particular emotions, processes, and levels of consciousness.[2] Peace, for example, is calibrated at 600 in contrast to guilt, which is a mere 30. If you feed your emotional body a steady diet of shame (20), despair (50) and regret (75), the average frequency of your diet is extremely low (48). Low frequency emotions are slow in vibration and "densify" your emotional body, weighing it down, causing obesity. At the same time, a starvation diet that deprives your emotional body can contribute to a feeble underweight condition or lead to bingeing on heavier, denser emotions in order to fill the void.

Light States

Level	Calibration
Peace	600
Joy	540
Compassion	500
Understanding	400
Forgiveness	350
Trust	250

Heavy States

Level	Calibration
Anger	150
Fear	100
Regret	75
Despair	50
Blame	30
Shame	20

Invoking and sustaining lighter feelings, faster in vibration, makes for a healthy emotional body. However, enacting higher frequency emotions is much easier said than done. This is often due to a misunderstanding of the emotional body and how it functions.

Information Not Plumbing

Based on physical models, the conventional wisdom tells us the emotional body needs to express. Its healing process is thought to parallel that of the physical body. If you cut your finger the wound bleeds and hurts for a while, but soon a scab forms, the pain subsides, and eventually the wound heals without a trace. The natural healing of the emotional body is thought to have similar stages: a sensation of discomfort or upset (the initial cut); emotional expression, which isn't always pretty (bleeding and scabbing); and completion (scab sloughing off). The emotional body's healing process is to express, but that process got interrupted by caregivers who forbade expression with messages of, "Don't cry. Don't be scared. Don't get mad," causing us to habitually hide or suppress our feelings. The repressed feelings were trapped inside, creating pressure that could best be equalized through uncovering and releasing, flushing them out. This approach has had limited success mostly because the emotional body is not a plumbing system; it's an energy/information system.

We now know that hormones, peptides, neurotransmitters, and receptor molecules that form the biochemical substance of the emotional body are *information based*.[3] Our body converts our emotions into molecular signals that get translated into cellular behavior. That means a key to dealing with emotions lies in shifting the signals, changing the frequencies.

Let's say you're heading down a crowded sidewalk, late for an appointment. Suddenly, you're bumped rather painfully from behind by someone who doesn't even apologize. You feel incensed. You turn around to give the person a piece of your mind and see the culprit is a little old man in a wheelchair, struggling to maneuver. Suddenly your anger vanishes without a trace. Where did it go? You internally reoriented yourself to the situation and your anger vanished. This recalibration is much like changing the channel on a television, or switching to a different frequency band on a cordless phone. The anger simply does not exist at your new frequency level.

There is no need to express or release the anger. Once you shift internal orientation, your entire system registers the new frequency and immediately recalibrates, right down to the cellular level.[4]

This transmutation may sound easy but I don't mean to oversimplify. There are many valid reasons why shifting frequencies doesn't always happen this way. One is the Amplifier Loop described above, in which the emotional and mental bodies get locked into a self-perpetuating pattern. With the wheelchair situation, shifting was easier because the old man was a stranger. The emotional reaction was more "pure" than, say, if you were jolted by someone you knew and didn't like.

Emotions are often kept in place by the stories we attach to them, a mixing of emotional and mental substance that predisposes us to Amplifier Loops. A second factor is that emotional inergies have a magnetic quality that causes them to self-attract, build up, and cluster together.[5] The magnetism of emotions contributes to emotional body cravings and addictions, discussed below. A third factor, already described, is a misunderstanding of the emotional body that perpetuates mistreatment of this body.

Suppression and Indulgence

Without proper education about emotional body needs, the tendency is either to suppress or indulge emotions. Both conditions are detrimental. First off, habitually trying to push away feelings doesn't work. A well-known study on suppression asked participants to avoid thoughts of a white bear while another group was allowed to think about anything, including

What we resist persists.

a white bear. The group who was asked to suppress thoughts actually ended up having more white bear thoughts than the free thinking group.[6] In the decades that followed, research on feeling and thought suppression shows the same results, which has been labeled "the rebound effect."[7] If you try to keep unpleasant feelings inside, you end up with more unpleasant feelings. Put another way, *what we resist persists.* The coagulated emotions can erect an inergetic barrier between yourself and others. Muffled emotions tend to grow and fester, clouding thinking and subduing all the emotions. If you try to quash anger or hurt, you can end up muting joy and tenderness as well. You can also predispose yourself to an emotional outburst when the proverbial last straw is added.

Not only is suppression bad for emotional body health, it is also physically harmful. Considerable inergy is needed to suppress emotions and that inergy is unavailable for other things, leading to an overall devitalized condition. Because of the close proximity of the physical and emotional bodies they interact and mutually influence each other. Habitually stuffing any emotion—especially anger—can be detrimental, even deadly. Suppression of emotion has been linked to everything from cancer, heart disease, arthritis, and high blood pressure to anorexia, bulimia, migraines and premature death.[8] Emotional suppression negatively impacts women more so than men, and the "cancer-personality" is characterized by chronically concealing unpleasant emotions behind a mask of cheerfulness.

At the same time, the over-expression of feelings is also harmful. It taxes the emotional body and stresses the physical. Emotional indulgence has been linked to a host of ills such as heart disease, high blood pressure, anxiety, depression, vision problems, gastro-intestinal problems, and migraines.[9] It has also been known to damage and destroy relationships.

Although there is no easy answer to the complexities of the emotional body, wisdom lies in the golden middle way: be aware of your feelings and attend to them when they are small. We will discuss this more, along with exercises, in the next chapter.

Before exploring the emotional body any further, let's take a look at yours. Complete the following checklist to learn more about the condition of your emotional body. Respond to each statement using your first impression without analyzing too much. There are no right or wrong answers. By answering as honestly as possible, you can discover more about your emotional body.

Your Emotional Body Type

Put an X next to each statement that applies to you.

_____ My feelings get hurt easily. (B)

_____ I am sensitive but not overly so. (A)

_____ Things just seem to roll off my back. (C)

_____ I cannot see a sad movie without crying. (B)

_____ When conflict arises, it's easy for me to stay rational. (C)

_____ I resolve conflict calmly when it comes up in my life. (A)

_____ I tend to take things personally. (B)

_____ I feel my feelings but they don't overtake me. (A)

_____ I have thick skin, nothing seems to bother me. (C)

_____ I sometimes wish I had thicker skin. (B)

_____ I almost never cry. (C)

_____ Friends tell me I am grounded and centered. (A)

_____ If an animal gets hurt or suffers I become very upset. (B)

_____ I stay in control in a crises. (C)

_____ If I am sad or angry I just state exactly that. (A)

_____ I sometimes wonder if I am depressed. (B)

_____ I try to stay upbeat and friendly. (C)

_____ Feelings are feelings, nothing more, nothing less. (A)

_____ My friends tell me to stop being so sensitive. (B)

_____ I can keep my cool when watching intense movies. (C)

_____ I feel good about my interactions with people. (A)

_____ When I get angry, my voice gets loud. (B)

_____ If there is a problem, I stay calm and figure it out. (C)

_____ I often disclose what I am feeling to those close to me. (A)

_____ I sometimes wish I didn't feel so much. (B)

_____ Friends tell me I am easy going. (C)

_____ I experience an array of mostly positive feelings. (A)

_____ I feel upset a lot of the time. (B)

_____ I almost never get angry. (C)

_____ I can tell you what I am feeling at any given moment. (A)

Scoring Your Results

Add up all your Xs and make a note of their corresponding letters.

Write your totals here:

_____ A   _____ B   _____ C

- **Most points A category**: You tend to have a healthy emotional body.

- **Most points in B category**: You tend to have an overweight emotional body.

- **Most points in C category**: You tend to have an underweight emotional body.

- **Points evenly distributed** among all three categories: Your emotional body tends toward weight fluctuations.

When the physical body suffers weight problems, it is prone to unhealthy eating habits, cravings, and food addictions. Similarly, the overweight emotional body has its own set of issues. In general, it is overly sensitive, reactive, prone to intensity, and addicted to drama. In contrast, the underweight emotional body is insensitive, under-active, prone to denial and addicted to avoidance. Let's look at the overweight condition first.

The Overweight Emotional Body

An overweight emotional body easily indulges. It lacks the self-discipline to pass up thrilling treats or heavy, fatty feelings. Emotions take on large proportions and are indulged in regularly.

Conditions of an overweight emotional body:

- Over-sensitive
- Reactive

- Prone to intensity
- Addicted to drama

If your emotional body is suffering from a weight problem you will find that you are overly sensitive to what people say. Your feelings frequently get hurt and the tendency is to take things personally. You may wish you had more control over this, hoping to let comments simply roll off your back. But try as you might, if you have a heavy emotional body, you will end up feeling upset and hurt a lot of the time. You will also be overly sensitive to other people's struggles. When friends talk about their problems you get upset as well, frequently taking sides, sticking up for your friend. You tend to feel the pain of others, which can be overwhelming.

Just as a pudgy physical body seeks out snacks, an oversized emotional body feeds on feelings and is quick to find them—and react—in any situation. With a bulky body, feelings are disproportionately big for the situation at hand. What others may register as a three on the emotional-intensity scale you experience as a ten. Because feelings loom so large, you have a hard time controlling them. They ramp up quickly, take over, and influence your behavior causing you to say or do things you may later regret.

In anticipation of a stressful conversation, for example, you may tell yourself you're not going to get upset. You might make it through the situation without over-reacting but afterwards find it hard to stop thinking about it. The overweight body is sluggish and digests slowly. An inordinate amount of time is spent processing emotional inergies. The emotions stay with you and eventually compel you to say something, if not to the person you are upset with, then to your friends who you emote with.

An overweight emotional body feasts on super-sized feelings. It likes to act out emotions with dramatic excess and has a hard time letting things go. If yours is obese, you'll experience roller-coaster rides of emotional intensity. Let's say a friend doesn't call and you feel hurt. Rather than simply saying, "I wish you had called when you said you would," and be done with it, your overweight body will enlarge the feeling and indulge it. Intoxicated by hurt, it may lead you to interrogate your friend and make it hard for you to listen. Or it can dictate that you fall silent and give the cold shoulder treatment. The obese body likes emotional intensity and can easily influence what you say and do.

An over-indulgent emotional body causes immobility. Instead of having an array of emotional expression, the overweight body is limited, constrained by its obesity. Usually one feeling-state predominates. This is most evident in times of stress. When life circumstances become challenging, the unwieldy body reacts in the same predictable way. The automatic response may be in the form of irritation or anxiety. However, it can even be a lighter emotion, like happiness, that shows up as incessant smiling or inappropriate laughter, masking the distress underneath. The key is not so much which one, but rather the presence of only one predominant feeling. Excess weight causes the body to become inflexible, so it reacts the same way to a variety of situations.

Just as an overweight physical body can suffer from food cravings, the overweight emotional body craves drama. There's an inability to tolerate long periods of calm. If emotional repose exists for too long, the overweight body needs a feelings-fix. This will drive it to whip up something to snack on or take other people's drama and use it for a quick emotional jolt. Taking other's drama requires a certain level of involvement in their affairs. In essence, the overweight body snitches other people's issues and claims them as its own. Much time is spent thinking about a friend or family member's problems, worrying and trying to figure them out as if they were its own. While you wouldn't think of swiping a loved one's belongings, others' problems are up for grabs often without you even noticing what you're doing. This is the sign of an emotional body suffering from drama addiction.

Addictions of the Overweight Emotional Body

In the case of the physical body, food addiction can play a major role in sabotaging any diet and perpetuating obesity. Certain foods lend themselves to addiction and they are usually foods that are harmful to our system. Have you ever heard of someone suffering from a broccoli or fresh spinach dependency? Sugar, saturated fat and carbohydrate addictions abound. Similarly, the emotional body is prone to addiction, and drama is its drug-of-choice.

What sugar is to the physical body, drama is to the emotional body. Sugar is added to an astonishing array of products in varied forms (i.e., white sugar, brown sugar, powdered sugar, sucrose, fructose, lactose, evaporated cane juice, corn syrup). Further, the physical body turns most carbohydrates into sugar. In like manner, drama is pervasive and the emotional body metabolizes many experiences into drama. Just as sugar comes in a variety of forms, so does drama.

The four most common drama derivatives are:

- Self-pity
- Hopelessness
- Alienation
- Guilt/Shame

A typical form drama takes is self-pity, a victim mentality in which life circumstances are seen as out of your control. When your emotional body is feeding on self-pity, you will be unable to see your part in things. You will tend to feel sorry for yourself and focus on the transgressions of others. Blind to your own behaviors, the world seems booby-trapped. You never know when a person or situation can turn on you. Instead of looking at your contribution to the issue, you are acutely aware of how others are mistreating you. Life circumstances, other people, even God, are conspiring to keep you down. The result is a pervasive "poor me" attitude that often invokes the sympathy of others, what notable self-help author Carolyn Myss has referred to as *woundology*.[10]

A second addiction of an overweight emotional body is hopelessness; the proverbial glass is always half empty. When met with life's difficulties, instead of rising to meet the challenge, the tendency is to lapse into despair. When your emotional body is feeding on hopelessness, an attitude of pessimism prevails. A common theme for those with this addiction is to focus on what's wrong in the world. You don't have to look very far to find problems and reasons to be overwhelmed. Self-talk is characterized by negative reminders: *there is no solution, it's useless, things will never change*. This, of course, nicely complements a self-pity addiction.

The third drama addiction is alienation. If your emotional body is feeding on alienation you often feel misunderstood. It's as if no one really "gets" you. With this addiction you believe you don't fit in; there's something strange about you that makes it impossible for you to feel comfortable, even in your own skin. You don't belong anywhere or with anyone. You are isolated and alone, unable to connect. No matter how hard you try, you are not seen or valued for who you are. In fact, you are often not seen at all, as feelings of invisibility prevail.

Another common emotional addiction is found in guilt/ shame. Inergetically speaking, these two feeling states are close enough to be interchangeable. The end result is the same: no matter what, it's your fault. You blame yourself and often feel haunted by perceived wrongdoing, unable to move on. Life events turn out as they do because you have some deficiency or defect. Self-talk is characterized by put-downs: *I'm not good enough, I did something wrong, I should have done better, it's my fault*. You are unable to resolve the situation by making amends or simply letting it go, as this would stop the guilt/shame. Since your emotional body is addicted, it must keep the supply coming.

Just as no two physical bodies are alike, every emotional body is unique. Drama addictions can take many forms. Although I have highlighted the major addictions and derivatives, this list is not exhaustive. Using self-pity, hopelessness, alienation and guilt/shame every once in a while does not constitute an addiction. However, if you find yourself indulging in them frequently, this is indicative of addiction. In the next chapter we will explore ways to break the cycle.

Emotional Body Junk Foods

An obese physical body is usually supported by favorite junk foods that contain some form of the addicted substance and are craved or binged on. Similarly, certain emotional junk foods have a high drama content and are craved by the overweight emotional body. Like a good chocolate spree, these treats tend to get indulged in repeatedly. The four most common emotional junk foods are:

- Fear
- Anger
- Gossip
- Irritation

Fear and anger top the emotional body junk food list because of their widespread use and availability in varied forms. Like most junk foods, fear and anger are socially sanctioned, mood-altering, and extremely satisfying in the moment. In addition, the biochemical cocktails they produce in the neighboring physical body are highly addictive.[11] This is a double-whammy that makes it even harder to stop using them. In the long run, the effects of overindulgence can be paralyzing as they contribute to emotional body obesity, and are then craved even more.

Another challenge of fear/anger junk foods is that they can pose as health food. They do this by presenting themselves as necessary for life. Anger self-talk usually goes something like this: *I have to be angry to be heard, to motivate others (or myself), to get things to change, to be strong or effective.* This sounds like a healthy and reasonable use of anger. But the truth is, you can be motivational, change-oriented, strong, and heard without indulging in anger, and your emotional body would be healthier.

Along the same lines, fear masks itself as a health food: *There are legitimate threats in the world and I have to be afraid to be prepared, to protect myself, and those I love.* This sounds essential for survival. There are valid concerns in life that we need to think about and prepare for. But fear is the tendency on the part of an overweight emotional body to inflate these to gain the maximum emotional stimulation. The truth is, you can be prepared and protected without indulging in fear.

Fear is sometimes diluted into worry that also masks itself as a health food. The self-talk goes something like this: *I worry because I care. If I don't worry it means I don't care. Therefore, I have to worry because this is important to me.* We want to think of ourselves as caring individuals but the truth is that worry and care are completely different

Emotional body junk foods pass as health foods.

inergetic frequencies. Worry wastes inergy by creating anxiety, a slow frequency, heavy emotion. Worry does not help a situation and can even make things worse by causing undue distress. Care, in contrast, is compassionate inergy. It carries with it feelings that are light and uplifting and produces loving actions. The key is in the inergy vibration of the feeling.

Another favorite junk food is gossip. The overweight emotional body thrives on using other people's problems for its own gratification, similar to a dessert fix for the sugar addict. Hours are spent, phone bills amassed, and endless cups of coffee consumed while the emotional body binges on gossip. In fact, so insatiable is this body's appetite for drama that gossip columns pervade newspapers, and entire publications are devoted to probing into the lives of celebrities to satisfy this craving. Supplying the addicted emotional body with gossip constitutes a billion dollar industry, a sad reflection on the severity of the problem.

Irritation is another favorite junk food that the overweight body enjoys. An addicted emotional body can turn just about anything into a quick irritation indulgence. The traffic, the co-workers, the food, the spouse, the kids, the dog—the opportunities are endless. Rather than representing a big dessert binge like fear, anger or gossip, irritation is more like little pieces of candy that are nibbled on throughout the day.

All four of the emotional body junk foods siphon off inergy. Much like sugar, some of them produce a jolting emotional high that is soon followed by a crash. Whether it's a junk food binge or a full-blown addiction, the common thread that runs through an overweight emotional body is drama, a pervasive problem for this body type. A drama addiction of any kind is de-inergizing in the long run.

In contrast to the overweight emotional body, the underweight emotional body has an aversion to drama. It is emotionally emaciated. This equally de-inergizing state carries its own set of challenges.

The Underweight Emotional Body

The underweight emotional body is almost allergic to emotions. If your emotional body is underweight, you will have an intolerance for feelings, particularly for the heavy, denser variety. Such expression will make you uncomfortable. Your frail emotional body is unaccustomed to a drama diet and is no match for an obese body. On a fundamental level, emotions themselves seem somehow threatening. But this may not prevent you from secretly snacking on emotional junk food at times.

Conditions of an underweight emotional body:

- Insensitive
- Under-active
- Prone to denial
- Addicted to avoidance

If your emotional body is underweight, you will tend to be insensitive to the emotional frequency band. Feelings are quite invisible—both yours and those of others. You often don't notice that you're emotionally affected by a situation until much later after an incident, if at all. A substantial time lag ensues and, in between, a lot of effort goes into convincing yourself that you shouldn't be upset. You tend to force yourself to think about other things. This doesn't address the issue so it just keeps coming back. You can be confused by its reappearance, and often wonder why people don't behave as you think they should.

An underdeveloped emotional body makes it hard to relate to the feelings of others. Their emotional expression seems foreign, as if they are speaking another language. Those around you seem to have exaggerated emotional reactions (which, by the way, they often must in order to get your attention emotionally). Being with a person who is emotionally upset is uncomfortable and undesirable. You tend to be at a loss for how to respond and feel awkward or fall silent as you try to figure it out. Since emotions are alien to you, they arouse suspicion: you think they may be used by others to manipulate you.

Under-activity characterizes the malnourished emotional body. The world could come to an end, it seems, and the emaciated emotional body would not respond because it is too starved to act. It passes off to the nearby physical and mental bodies and lets them do all the work. To protect a fragile emotional body, often an invisible wall gets erected in which nothing can pass through. No emotion is let in or out. This causes the emotional body to become rigid and to react in the same way to any of life's challenges. No matter what happens, you consistently appear calm, even cheerful, on the outside. But inside is a different story.

With an underweight emotional body, feelings are often confusing and overwhelming, therefore, best to be avoided. You tend to deny your own feelings as well, which includes denying any emotionally-based needs and wants. You'd rather not be bothered with all the turmoil. But by denying feelings, life becomes dull and monotonous. In starving your emotional body, the entire spectrum of feelings becomes unavailable. With no joy, enthusiasm, or empathy you often feel like a robot, just going through the motions while feeling hollow and vacant inside.

The underweight emotional body does not suffer from the array of drama cravings that the obese body does. However, it is not immune to addiction. Underweight addiction takes the form of avoidance—emotions are habitually avoided. They are seen as messy (unnecessary, irrelevant, even dangerous) and therefore not to be paid attention to. The logic goes: *The more you pay attention to your feelings, the more unruly they get. They should be downplayed. If you are upset about something, just focus on something else and the upset will go away.* This may work at times, but as a general mode of being it leads to the habitual avoidance of feelings. Consequently, the emotional body is starved of emotional inergy. Since none is available, it feeds off of the bodies next to it—the physical and mental. The avoidance addiction takes two forms. If the mental body is involved, the result is a rationalization addiction. With the physical body, it's an activity addiction.

If you suffer from rationalization addiction, you habitually use your mental body to explain away unacceptable behaviors or feelings and avoid the truth. Instead of looking at your role in things, you devise logical, plausible explanations that justify your behavior. Your mental body becomes fueled by the vacuum created from an emaciated emotional body. This inergy vortex super-charges your mental body and makes it adept at calculating ironclad explanations about how things should be and why you are not at fault. You probably like to argue and, predictably, you win. However, never admitting a mistake, it's almost impossible to grow and change.

If you have an activity addiction, you will use tasking and "busy-ness" to avoid feeling or dealing with undesirable emotions. A vacuous emotional body fuels your physical body and you are predisposed to endless activity. This can take the form of workaholism, time-consuming projects around the house, excessively demanding physical fitness regimes, or a constantly filled social calendar. Doing-ness is used to avoid feeling.

Whether it's avoidance addiction, insensitivity, or denial, the thread that runs through the underweight emotional body involves under-functioning on the emotional level and over-functioning on the physical or mental. Individuals with this condition often display android behavior, especially in personal conflicts. They seem emotionally anorexic and flat. Instead of having dynamic emotional inergies, the underweight body is deficient.

The under- and overweight conditions represent opposite poles on a spectrum of possibilities. Chances are your emotional body is somewhere in between. It's also possible to fluctuate from one extreme to the other in an effort to attain balance. Similar to crash dieting, a chronically overweight body may gain short-term benefit from going temporarily underweight, and vice versa. You probably find that you behave overweight in some situations and underweight in others. This body is not static but quite changeable depending on the situation. When your emotional body interacts with the bodies of others it is affected by them as well.

The Healthy Emotional Body

A healthy emotional body is fit and proportionate to your overall inergy constitution. Emotions are seen as messengers of inergies from the emotional plane. They are received, decoded, and acted upon in a conscious manner that involves choice instead of automatic reactions. In general, a healthy emotional body is:

- Sensible
- Compassionate
- Resilient
- Pure

If your emotional body is healthy, you have achieved a high degree of sensibility. You are able to sense things on the emotional level with a savvy perceptibility. This is not to be confused with the hyper-sensitivity of the obese body in which there is over-reaction and a predisposition to take things personally. Instead, sensibility means having the ability to be aware of and discern the subtleties of the emotional body. You take *in* but do not take *on* emotional inergies. The channel is open but not exaggerated. You apprehend feelings and do so without the avoidance of the underweight body and without the excesses of the obese body indulging emotions, making them bigger.

This type of sensibility involves the mental body but is not to be confused with the hyper-functioning of the mental as in the case of the underweight body. A healthy emotional body is able to cooperate with the mental body and accept its assistance in interpretation of emotional inergies. There is not the leeching of mental inergy caused by a starved emotional body. In a healthy body this assistance takes the form of a mutually beneficial co-working between the two. The emotional body senses emotional inergies in a neutral manner—its own as well as others—and the mental body assists in discernment and interpretation of the inergy input. Emotions are simply seen for what they are—inergy—nothing more and nothing less. They are witnessed and observed in a matter-of-fact way. You see them as signals that condition experience much like the weather conditions the day. You then decode and respond to those signals with compassion for yourself and others.

> You take *in* but don't take *on* emotional inergies.

The emotional body links us to others on a feeling level. It allows us to have sympathy, kindness, and empathy. However, this is not the kind of empathy in which you take on other people's emotions, as the overweight body is inclined to do. If your emotional body is healthy you are compassionate toward others, considerate of their circumstances, while allowing them to take responsibility for themselves. You respond with love and care without taking on their issues and without enabling their emotional cravings or addictions. You care for your own body by abstaining from emotional addictions and junk foods and cultivating compassion. Self-inducing compassion is shown to have beneficial effects, not only for the emotional body, but for the mental and physical as well.[12]

A healthy emotional body is fresh, clean, and current to the present moment. Emotions are pure and innocent, so to speak. They are not covered up by an arsenal of defenses, protected by self-righteousness, steely indifference, or a wall of exuberance. Instead, feelings are easily accessed in their pure form. Disappointment is disappointment. Irritation is irritation. Happiness is happiness. They are not conglomerates of feelings—hurt mixed with fearful memories covered over by a thick layer of hostility and blame. They are experienced and expressed in their untainted form.

Unlike the rigidity of the under- and overweight emotional bodies, your healthy emotional body experiences a dynamic array of varied feeling states on the lighter side of the inergy scale. That's because you acknowledge feelings when they are small. They don't have to get big and intense in order to be noticed, nor do you over-indulge them. They are self-observed when they are subtle and attended to. The healthy body is not starved of emotional inergy nor is it contaminated by junk foods. There is no backlog of repressed emotions, no holding on to things, no outbursts or over-expression. Instead, you are in touch with the content of your body and attending to it as an open channel of energy and information.

With a healthy emotional body, you respond to life's circumstances instead of over- or under-reacting. You do not engage in automatic behaviors; you are free to choose your response. You are in control and responsible; you are "response-able." In any given moment, you are able to respond to a situation in the best possible way. Your healthy emotional body is supple and adaptive to any circumstances. It is resilient: simultaneously strong and flexible.

In the next chapter we explore specific steps to a healthy emotional body, learning ways to help it become more balanced, along with exercises to sustain it.

Chapter Six

Steps to a Healthy Emotional Body

Kate recently discovered a lump in her right breast. Her latest mammogram had shown nothing and she knew that being pre-menopausal often causes changes in breast tissue. She didn't want to get alarmed but scheduled a doctor appointment right away, just to be on the safe side. After the examination, he recommended she have another mammogram. Kate had already had two and dreaded the thought of another. Knowing that mammograms are painful and would expose her to more cancer causing radiation, she was reluctant. She had recently heard about another early detection method, thermography, that she was told is safe, painless, and more effective. She mentioned to her doctor that she would rather do breast thermography. He flatly replied, "If you want to be your own doctor then you don't need me," and left the room. Kate felt alone and confused.

* * *

Allison knew that Ben's daughter from a previous marriage was visiting. This was the first time his five-year-old was able to visit him alone, without her mom. Allison wanted to be a supportive friend, so she invited father and daughter for a sailboat ride at a nearby lake. She had planned to pick them up at ten. However, at the last minute she realized that because of Memorial Day the boats would be in demand by families on holiday. She called Ben at 8:30 that morning and suggested they leave half an hour earlier. He didn't answer so she left a message. He called back at nine, obviously flustered, and lectured her about how he couldn't possibly move any faster and why did she expect them to rush around on such short notice. Allison felt defensive and began to wonder why she invited them in the first place. The outing was tainted.

* * *

By all accounts, at the age of 53 Jeremy had crafted the perfect life. His happy marriage, bright and well-adjusted children, profitable company, and social life were all thriving. His health was nearly optimal too. It'd been a full year since a successful surgery to remove a cancerous prostate. Although his sexual ability had not returned, he remained 100% cancer free. Yet, for mysterious reasons, he had started waking up in the middle of the night stricken with anxiety and despair that seemed to have no point of origin and no correlation to his happy life. The feelings pervaded for weeks and the lack of sleep made it hard to function. Jeremy was baffled by his irrational behavior but couldn't stop it.

* * *

Each of these stories demonstrates the impact of an unhealthy emotional body. The result is often confusion, anxiety, distraction, and stressful misunderstandings. Unfortunately, situations like these are all too familiar. A healthy emotional body is a rare occurrence. We tend to either deprive or indulge this body because we simply don't know how to deal with its forceful inergies. When we feel anxious, depressed, or irritable, we may attribute our discomfort to external influences—other people, a need to get away, physical ailments, or a bad day. This doesn't make the feelings go away and can even compound them. We may do nothing, which can cause us to isolate and decline into deeper distress.

One in four Americans[1] and nearly half of young people suffer some sort of mental health disorder.[2] If professional help is sought, it usually involves psychiatric medication, an increasingly profitable business. Although the data are hard to come by, in 2002 drug companies made $12 billion in profits from antidepressants alone, mostly from increasing use on infants and children.[3] The sales of many companies have tripled in the interim. These are troubling numbers. Inergy health education and caring for the emotional body have never been more urgent.

Emotional Body Hygiene

A little over 70 years ago in the US, the Red Cross was canvassing the country teaching home hygiene and care of the sick. They taught disease prevention techniques such as sanitizing water and food, hand washing, and proper disposal of waste that are now second nature. Many elaborate time-consuming rituals currently get enacted in an effort to care for the physical body. We take our temperature, do blood pressure readings, exercise regularly, stock up on vitamins, and assess calories and cholesterol. But the emotional body is chronically neglected. The path to a healthy emotional body must start at the level of basic hygiene. By paying attention and doing fundamental hygiene you can help insure your body gets its basic needs met. Whether yours is underweight, overweight, or suffers weight fluctuations, all three conditions can be helped by emotional body hygiene.

Developing your inner senses is the key to emotional body health and the focus of the exercises that follow. They include simple hygiene, basic treatments, and advanced techniques. It's important that the exercises be followed in order. If your physical body were injured or ill, you wouldn't rush off to the nearest gym and attempt a rigorous training program. Similarly, jumping from long term emotional body neglect to advanced training with nothing in between is unwise. If you skip the hygiene and basic treatment steps below, you can strain your emotional body by subjecting it to too much too soon.

Take Responsibility

Most of us were raised with exclusive focus on our physical and intellectual wellbeing. A parent's duty was to put a roof over your head, food on the table, and send you to a good school. No attention was paid to emotional development. Schools, as well, were only concerned with educating the mental and physical bodies. There was no such thing as emotional literacy. Thanks to emotional intelligence proponent Daniel Goleman,[4] this is starting to change in some locations with emotional literacy and behavioral health classes now introduced into the elementary and secondary school curricula. Those of us who missed this education have some catching up to do.

A good place to start is to realize that your emotional bodily functions are your own. This sounds obvious but in practice it's not. We habitually try to make others responsible for our own emotions. The pervasive belief is that other people make us feel things. This is most evident in how feelings are talked about.

Request instead of complain or criticize.

By saying things like, "You make me so mad," or, "You scared me," and, "You hurt me," your own emotional experience gets attributed to someone else, effectively turning feelings into fault.

When you assign your emotions to other people, you are putting others in control of your emotional body. When you fault others for what you are feeling, it's the equivalent of saying, "You make me have the hiccups," or "You made my leg cramp." We would never say that because it sounds absurd; we know it's not true. We know we are responsible for our physical body functioning. We would not say, "You make me imagine the crowded freeway," or "You make me think of the cloth napkin." We acknowledge that we are responsible for our own thoughts and physical functions; it's time to take responsibility for our emotions as well.

Taking responsibility means recognizing that you have an emotional body and that you determine your emotional experience. Your emotions are yours. Other people do not make you feel things.

You react the way you do because of your emotional constitution. Someone else would react in another way because theirs is different. You feel things because your unique emotional body gives you the capacity to register inergies on the emotional channel of experience in your particular way. Rather than falsely attribute your emotional experience to others, claim it as your own. A good place to start is by changing how you talk about feelings. Replace you-language with I-language. Instead of, "You hurt me," or "You make me mad," take ownership of your emotional body by saying, "I feel hurt," or "I am angry," and so forth.

Another way to take responsibility for your emotional body is to request instead of criticize or complain. Ask for what you want rather than faulting the other person for not giving it to you. Let's say your daughter doesn't make her bed on a regular basis and this irritates you. The tendency would be to say to her, "You never make your bed," which is a complaint, at best, or a criticism, at worst. You feel irritated and are, in effect, making your daughter responsible for those feelings. Instead, turn your complaint into a request, "I'd like you to make your bed each morning." This allows you to stay constructive and own your feelings by asking for what you want to improve the situation. Maybe you notice that your partner has been very busy at work and you're feeling sad and neglected. Instead of saying, "Seems like you never want to do anything anymore," which can sound blaming, try "I'd love it if we could go out later this week." This simple turn of phrase can make a big difference between a defensive reaction and a favorable response. Take responsibility for what you are feeling, speak in I-statements (omit the you), and ask for what you want.

Exercise: Take Responsibility
Application: Ongoing, to take responsibility for your emotional body
Time: Instantaneous

- When you are talking about your feelings, refrain from attributing your emotions to another person. Instead, speak in I-statements, claiming your emotions as your own.

- Ask for what you want instead of complaining or criticizing.

Emotional Body Mirror Check

In order to assess our physical body, we observe it. *Are my hands clean? Do I look fat?* We examine it by looking in a mirror. *Is there food between my teeth? Do I need to comb my hair?* We wouldn't think of being seen in public without first doing a quick mirror check and making changes accordingly. Yet we habitually interact with others without having self-observed our emotional body. For hygienic reasons, it's important to assess your emotional body on an ongoing basis so you can make minor adjustments before conditions get too extreme. The following exercise is a self-observation check-in for the emotional body.

Exercise: Emotional Body Mirror Check
Application: At least once a day, to assess the condition of your emotional body
Time: 1-2 minutes

- Find a quiet place in which you can focus without distraction.

- Be as physically comfortable as possible.

- Take a couple of slow, deep breaths.

- Close your eyes and intentionally shift your attention away from an external focus toward an internal focus, awakening your internal senses.

- In your mind's eye, see a mirror in front of you. Instead of your physical body, this mirror is reflecting your emotional body.

- Notice everything you can about your emotional body. How does it look today? What color is it? Shape? Size? What stands out? Notice the details. Anything you need to adjust? Overall condition?

- Whenever this feels complete, open your eyes.

If you discover that your body is in need of adjustment, use the exercises that follow to address the needs accordingly.

Label and Let Go

Just as thoroughly cleaning your physical body is necessary for personal hygiene, so is carefully cleaning your emotional body. Emotions are the substance of this body so keeping it clean requires focusing on feelings, the whole spectrum, including those you may not want to look at or talk about. It seems we all want to be happy but when it comes to unpleasant feelings we want nothing to do with them. We embrace the emotional body when it's feeling good and reject it when it deviates from that, hoping the unwanted feelings will just go away. But emotions are inergy and inergy does not go away. It can, however, be transformed from one frequency to another.

One of the ways to transform emotional inergy is through the use of feeling-words. The act of labeling emotions with words has been shown to produce therapeutic effects in the brain.[5] When you shift from *sensing* an emotion to *observing* the emotion enough to label it with a word, your brain reconfigures and the emotion dissipates. However, not just any word will do; the emotion must be labeled with a word that identifies the emotion (i.e., hurt, afraid). This involves switching from self-sensing to self-observation. Using unrelated words or more generic terms does not produce the therapeutic effects.

The exercise below is helpful for the overweight body because labeling emotions in words shifts inergy away from the emotional body and engages the mental. It's a self-talk exercise that, with practice, can be done in the moment to help diffuse emotional inergy. It strengthens and develops your inner senses, your ability to shift between self-sensing and self-observing. Done on an ongoing basis, the exercise also helps to transform feelings when they are small. Bringing attention to feelings when they are subtle prevents the intensity that often results in high drama. Once the body is cleaned, the exercise helps maintain overall hygiene by giving the emotional body the ongoing care and attention it needs. It is appropriate for all body types.

The exercise is also beneficial for the underweight body because it helps this body end its avoidance addiction. The exercise involves getting in touch with feelings, something the underweight emotional body is not accustomed to doing. We know that maintaining physical health requires movement of the body. If you become sedentary your physical body deteriorates. Similarly, the emotional body requires movement or it atrophies. Like the physical, the emotional body responds very well to exercise, which consists of the movement of feelings. The exercise also helps end a rationalization addiction because it requires the underweight body to bring attention to emotions, connecting the intellect with the feelings, creating an inergetic bridge between the emotional and mental bodies.

Those with an underweight emotional body may find the exercise challenging at first. The habitual denial of feelings that characterizes an underweight condition can make accessing feelings arduous. If you attempt the exercise and find it too strenuous, try waking up your atrophied emotional muscle by focusing on your abdomen where your solar plexus center, the seat of emotion, is located. Focus your attention in that area and set your intent to self-sense your feelings. Breathe into your solar plexus and use self-talk to affirm that you can now safely feel your feelings. If you stay with the exercise over time, the emotional muscle reengages and you will find it progressively easier to be aware of feelings.

The exercise that follows involves using four basic feeling categories of *mad, sad, scared, and glad.*[6] These are meant as broad umbrella terms under which a variety of feelings can fit. You may be telling yourself that you don't get mad; it's too extreme. But milder forms of anger are also included under the basic category. Most feelings can be condensed down to, or are combinations of, the four basic emotions. Feeling irritated, annoyed, angry, frustrated, resentful, and enraged are all variations of feeling mad. Feeling disappointed, depressed, guilty, ashamed, hurt, or hopeless can be distilled down to sadness. Feeling nervous, anxious, afraid, worried, shy, terrified, and panicky can be traced to fear. Feelings of joy, happiness, excitement, compassion, or appreciation are related to gladness. Be sure to repeat the feeling word in front of each new item:

- *I am mad about (insert item 1 here).*
- *I am mad about (insert item 2 here).*
- *I am mad about (insert item 3 here).*

The exercise starts with *mad* and finishes with *glad* so the emotional body is experiencing a higher frequency inergy at the end of the exercise. You may find the *glad* category to be easier than the previous three. If your emotional body is fit and vitalized there are likely many things you are glad about. If your emotional body is stressed, you may find it hard to come up with happy things. Give yourself time and do your best.

Although the exercise may be done as a journaling activity with your responses written down, this is not recommended. It's meant to be a self-talk activity. The purpose of naming emotions in words is to transform them. The exercise is a cleaning process and, just as you wouldn't capture your dirty bath water to preserve it, you probably don't want to hold on to your old emotions by writing them down. It's better to sort through them, label them in words, and let them go.

Exercise: Label and Let Go
Application: At least once a week, to clean the emotional body and transform feelings.
Time: Varies, depending on the emotional body's condition (approx. 5-15 minutes)

- Find a quiet place in which you can focus without distraction.

- Be in a seated position, as comfortable as possible.

- Take a couple of slow, deep breaths.

- Gently close your eyes and intentionally shift your attention away from an external focus toward an internal focus, using your intent to tune in to your emotional body.

- Using self-talk, you are about to ask and answer a question. Formulate the words in your mind.

- The question is: *What am I mad about?*

- Allow the things you are mad about to come to mind, one at a time (i.e., *I am mad about the dirty house. I am mad about being so far behind in my work*, etc). Say them one by one. Look for anger in any form, big upsets or tiny irritations. This is not a time for problem solving or ruminating. Just call to mind each thing you are mad about and move on to the next. Stay with the process until you run out of anger items. Then move on to the next category.

- *What am I sad about?*

- Allow all of the things you are sad about to come to mind, one after the other. Look for sadness in any form (disappointment, depression, guilt, shame, hopelessness). Again, this is not a time for brainstorming solutions or going into the problem. Just call to mind what you are sad about, label each thing (*I am sad about . . .*), and continue with your list. When you have run out of things you are sad about move on to the next category.

- *What am I scared about?*

- Allow all of the things you are scared about to come to mind, one after the other. Look for fear in any form (anxiety, nervousness, shyness, panic). Just call to mind what you are scared about, label each thing (*I am scared about . . .*) and continue listing them. When you have run out of things you are scared about move on to the last category.

- *What am I glad about?*

- Look for gladness in any form (joy, happiness, excitement, gratitude, enthusiasm, appreciation). Allow all of the things you are glad about to come to mind, one after the other.

- Whenever this feels complete you can open your eyes.

The Label and Let Go exercise is a cleaning process designed to help you find, name, and thereby transform emotions through words. You can enact this as a self-talk exercise in the moment, much like a mindfulness practice, to label and let go of feelings in day-to-day situations.

Basic Treatments

Once emotional body hygiene is in place, you can move on to a more advanced program of basic treatments. Remember, treatments do not replace hygiene. You still need to wash your body as any treatment techniques will work better on a clean body. Our health treatment kit for the emotional body contains Assurance, Tapping, and Reversals.

Assurance

Sometimes cleaning your body isn't enough. Your skin can become dry, flaky, and minor abrasions get easily inflamed. You would use body lotion or ointment to protect your skin from the elements. Lotion for the emotional body takes the form of reassuring self-talk. The ointment of assurance should be applied liberally and regularly.

Assurance requires that you discern what is going on with your emotional body and speak words of affirmation and comfort to it. It is a salve applied specifically to the emotional body and must be understood within this context. Assurance is not meant to solve the problem. Its purpose is to address the emotional body's needs and protect it from inflammation. Once emotional arousal is prevented, you return to the problem at hand. You will be able to deal with life's challenges much more effectively if your emotional body is soothed and supple.

The following situations illustrate the difference between emotional assurance versus inflammation. Before reading these situations take a moment to awaken your emotional body so that you can sense into the emotional content of each response. Allow your emotional body to be primary and your mental body to stay in the background, being careful not to comment on the responses with your intellect. Instead, use self-sensing to discern how each response would *feel emotionally*. Put a plus (+) next to the response that feels soothing and a minus (-) next to the response that feels emotionally stressful.

> **Situation**: You have a heated argument with your fiancé that doesn't end well.

> _____ Response #1: You tell yourself it's over; you just wasted the last ten months of your life. You'd better cut your losses and start making contingency plans.

> _____ Response #2: You tell yourself that everything will be alright, that you have worked through difficulties before and you'll get through this one as well, together.

> **Situation**: You make a mistake and the boss snaps at you.

> _____ Response #1: You fear for your job, telling yourself that you really blew it this time.

> _____ Response #2: You tell yourself it was a small mistake and the rest of your work is exemplary; the boss was probably having a bad day and the mistake will likely be forgotten by tomorrow.

> **Situation**: Your adolescent yells at you to leave her alone.

> _____ Response #1: You blame her, telling yourself she is over-reactive and defiant.

_____ Response #2: You tell yourself that she is a good kid who is doing her best. She's allowed to have a little flare-up. You can ask her about it later if need be.

Situation: You're late for an appointment.

_____ Response #1: You anticipate scornful looks and unpleasant consequences.

_____ Response #2: You tell yourself that you will arrive in good time, others have run late in the past, and people will be glad to see you.

The second responses are reassuring and the first are inflammatory. If you are like most people, the second responses are much more soothing to your emotional body than the first. Also, like most people, the first responses probably sound quite familiar. Again, assurance is not about rationalizing mistakes or denying the issue. The purpose of it is to calm the emotional body so you can address the issue without unnecessary emotional charge.

Exercise: Assurance
Application: As needed, apply liberally to sooth and comfort the emotional body
Time: Instantaneous

- Whenever you find yourself stressed, use your intent along with affirming self-talk to sooth and comfort your emotional body.

It's important to apply the ointment of assurance right away; quick application prevents inflammation and infection. Assurance also works for others. If you interact with someone whose emotional body is inflamed, you can apply the ointment of assurance to their emotional body as well by saying soothing statements.

Tapping

Sometimes after Assurance the emotional body is still in need. The situation was too painful or the emotional body too vulnerable. You find yourself dealing with feelings that don't seem to be addressed by basic hygiene or Assurance. Further intervention is needed. Tapping is helpful, especially for an overweight body. It transforms emotional inergies and also works to interrupt Amplifier Loops where resonant inergies in the emotional and mental bodies self-perpetuate (described in Chapter 5).

The technique below is an adaptation of the Emotional Freedom Technique (EFT)[7] that uses tapping a series of acupoints on the skin as its basis. The process is amazingly simple yet powerfully effective. Five million people worldwide use EFT with positive results for a variety of issues such as anxiety, depression, and improved athletic performance. EFT emerges from an exciting new field of energy psychology in which inergy interventions show great promise where other methods fall short. For example, Post-Traumatic Stress Disorder (PTSD) is one of the most difficult emotional traumas to treat, affecting tens of thousands of war veterans. Yet preliminary studies with Iraq vets dealing with PTSD show a 50% drop in PTSD after EFT treatment (in sometimes as few as six sessions); follow-up shows that one year after treatment reduced stress levels are sustained.[8]

Tapping acupoints is an effective way of transforming emotional inergies and recalibrating the emotional body. The tapping exercise may look strange but the effects are profound. The acupoints are part of the vital/physical interface (the Interface Effect was described in Chapter 3). As such, they represent a gateway between the emotional and physical bodies and can remix the bio-chemical-inergetic cocktails that often drive our system. There are a variety of tapping sequences that work. We'll use a three-step process outlined below. More information about each step, variations, and details of how the process works are available elsewhere.[9] Our purpose is to learn a basic technique and use it to help the emotional body.

Step 1: The Set-Up

In the tapping sequence, particular phrases are used concurrently while tapping. These set-up phrases are specific to the emotional issue you're dealing with. Stimulating the acupoints while speaking certain words effectively encodes the new energy/ information into your system.[10] Devising the best set-up phrase is a three-step process.

First, think about the emotionally upsetting situation and do your best to formulate the issue into words. It may be something like this:

- *I am disappointed in my daughter.*

- *I cannot forgive my mother.*

- *I resent my irresponsible roommate.*

- *I am so lazy and pathetic.*

- *I am hurt beyond belief by my insensitive partner.*

Second, plug your issue into a format in which you are talking about the issue, and then affirm that you love and accept yourself anyway. Here is the format: *Even though I have this (insert issue here) I deeply and completely accept myself.* Altering your words so that you are talking *about* the issue (i.e., I *have* disappointment versus I *am* disappointed) shifts your perspective to a more objective stance. You are no longer *in* the feeling; you are *observing* it. It shifts attention—and therefore inergy—away from your emotional body and into your mental body. This shift from self-sensing to self-observation helps transform the emotional inergy of the issue and anchor the inergy in self-compassion. Using the sample issues above, the final phrases would be like this:

- *Even though I have this disappointment in my daughter, I deeply and completely accept myself.*

- *Even though I have this inability to forgive my mother, I deeply and completely accept myself.*

- *Even though I have this resentment for my roommate, I deeply and completely accept myself.*

- *Even though I have this belief that I am lazy and pathetic, I deeply and completely accept myself.*

- *Even though I have this hurt, I deeply and completely accept myself.*

Third, the phrase is repeated while stimulating karate-chop points, the part of your hand you would use to deliver a karate chop (see Figure 6.1). This is the fleshy part of the outside of each hand beneath the little fingers. You can do both of the karate-chop points at the same time by "clapping" your hands together at those points, as though you were "karate chopping" your hands.

Step 2: The Tapping Sequence

The phrases are repeated while tapping nine sets of points at specific locations on the body (Figure 6.1). These correspond to acupoints points that have been shown to correct disruptions in the vital body that accompany charged emotional states. (The lips and collar points are the same as in the Collar+Lips+Tail exercise from Chapter 4). The points are located on both sides of the body. Although, technically speaking, you could tap just one side of the body, tapping both sides is more thorough. Each point should be tapped about five to seven times each with your fingertips using medium pressure.

TAPPING PROCEDURE

#1... THE SETUP

Repeat 3X: "*Even though I have this (problem),
I deeply and completely accept myself*" while
continuously tapping the Karate Chop point.

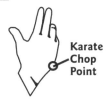

Karate
Chop
Point

#2... THE SEQUENCE
Tap about 5X on each point

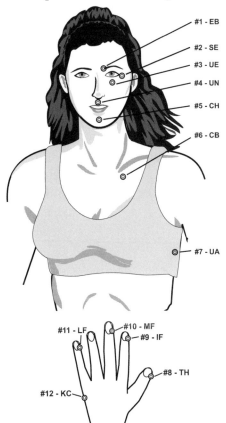

#1 - EB
#2 - SE
#3 - UE
#4 - UN
#5 - CH
#6 - CB
#7 - UA
#11 - LF
#10 - MF
#9 - IF
#8 - TH
#12 - KC

#3... THE GAMUT
Perform 9 actions while
tapping the Gamut Point
continuously:

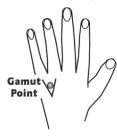

Gamut
Point

1) Eyes closed
2) Eyes open
3) Eyes hard down right
   (head steady)
4) Eyes hard down left
   (Head steady)
5) Roll eyes in a circle
6) Roll eyes in opposite
   direction
7) Hum 5 seconds of song
   (Happy Birthday)
8) Count from 1 to 5
9) Hum 5 seconds of a
   song again.
End by tapping the Karate
Chop Point.

Figure 6.1 The 3 steps of the Tapping exercise.
(Graphic by Gwenn Bonnell. Used with kind permission.)

The points are:

1. Beginning of the eyebrows
2. Sides of the eyes
3. Under the eyes
4. Under the nose
5. Under the lower lip
6. Under the collar bones
7. Under the arms, on the side of the rib cage
8. On the tip of each finger/thumb except the ring finger
9. Karate-chop points

Step 3: The Gamut Point

The exercise ends with tapping what is called the *gamut* point on the back of each hand, between the little finger and ring finger knuckle, about half an inch toward the wrist (see Figure 6.1). While tapping this point, nine actions are performed. Most of the actions consist of eye movements that are shown to stimulate certain areas of the brain that reinforce the inergy shift.[11] Humming and counting involve both the left (counting) and right (humming) brain hemispheres. The nine actions are:

1. Eyes closed
2. Eyes open
3. Eyes down sharp right
4. Eyes down sharp left
5. Roll eyes in a complete circle
6. Roll eyes in a circle in the opposite direction
7. Hum five seconds of a song (i.e., Happy Birthday)
8. Count from one to five
9. Hum five seconds of a song again

With practice, the entire sequence can be done in less than three minutes. It's best to start and end the exercise with self-sensing your emotional body. If the emotional charge seems not to transform enough, repeat the exercise until it does.

Exercise: Tapping
Application: As needed, for larger issues of the emotional body. Especially helpful for overweight conditions and for interrupting Amplifier Loops.
Time: 3 minutes

- Self-sense your emotional body to assess the level of emotional intensity.

- Form a phrase regarding the emotionally charged issue: *Even though I have this (insert issue here) I deeply and completely accept myself.*

- Stimulate karate-chop points while repeating your phrase.

- Tap eyes, lips, collar, underarms, fingertips, and karate-chop points while repeating your phrase.

- Tap the gamut point while doing the eye movements and hum, count, hum.

- Self-sense your emotional body to assess the level of emotional intensity.

- Repeat the exercise until the intensity dissipates.

Inergy Reversal

Sometimes you find yourself dealing with emotions that need a different type of treatment. Maybe you are in the middle of a conversation in which you get emotionally activated and doing the tapping would not be appropriate. Maybe you don't have time to do the tapping. In contrast, the reversal exercise can be done anytime, anywhere. It consists of acting the opposite of what your emotional body is feeling. It is used when your body is running heavy emotions (i.e., anything in the fear or anger categories). If, say, your staff member is not performing and you're annoyed with her, about to launch into criticism, instead of snapping at her, do the opposite. Compliment her on something she does well (hopefully you can find at least one thing in that red-hot moment). Then later, after your emotional charge has transformed, you can talk about her poor performance without your irritation contaminating the conversation.

A reversal can also work immediately after the fact. Let's say you're annoyed and just criticized your staff. You can immediately follow the criticism with a reversal, meaning, giving compliments or praise. This will help transform your low frequency annoyance in the moment as well as help your staff feel better. Again, you may need to have a follow-up conversation in which the performance issue gets addressed without the emotional charge impacting the conversation. The potency of the emotional body requires special attention. This body should not be allowed to overtake a conversation, as it wants to do, especially in an overweight condition.

Doing the opposite of what you are feeling may sound like suppression but it is not. Suppression stops the inergy flow and drives powerful emotional inergy deeper into your system, where it often manifests physically. In contrast, a reversal simply reverses the *information* on an inergy channel without stopping the *energy* flow. It does this by decoupling the information from the energy. It's especially helpful for an overweight condition because it transforms emotional inergies and engages the mental body. It also interrupts Amplifier Loops.

Enacting the opposite of what your emotional body is feeling can be difficult, especially when the intensity level is high. The reversal will feel artificial, insincere, uncomfortable, even forced. If you experience any of these you are doing the exercise correctly. The biggest obstacle to a successful reversal is the misconception that it's inauthentic. True, the reversal is not authentic to your emotional body because you're asked to do the opposite of what you're feeling. However, oftentimes it *is* authentic to your other bodies, and their needs are equally valid. When your emotional body is misbehaving, so to speak, it should not be allowed to have its way. Being exclusively authentic to your emotional body in highly charged situations usually happens at the expense of the other bodies. This is why we end up saying or doing things we later regret. To avoid this, we must take all the bodies into account and not let an inflamed emotional body rule the day. Reverse the information but let the energy flow. Of course, ideally, we want to act as a whole, and act with compassion, having the information and the energy aligned. However, in the meantime: *fake it till you make it.*

> **Exercise: Inergy Reversal**
> Application: As needed, for larger issues of the emotional body. Especially helpful for overweight conditions and for interrupting Amplifier Loops.
> Time: Instantaneous
>
> * When you are running heavy or intense emotions and you want to interrupt the pattern, speak or act the opposite of what your emotional body is feeling.

With due diligence, even intense emotional habits can be successfully transformed. Coupled with Assurance and Tapping, this completes the basic emotional body treatment kit. Once this program has been mastered, you are ready for advanced techniques to boost your immunity and take your emotional body to the next level.

Advanced Techniques

The steps to a healthy emotional body progress in order. It's important not to skip hygiene or basic health treatments and jump into advanced techniques. These techniques are to be done when the emotional body has attained a certain degree of health. In other words, you have been practicing the hygiene and basic techniques outlined above on an ongoing basis and feel relatively emotionally healthy. If you attempt immune strengthening without having a strong foundation to build on, not only will the strengthening not work, you risk compromising your emotional body.

Immune Strengthening

Immune strengthening involves training the emotional body to be resilient in the face of strong emotional inergies and red-hot moments of intensity. This requires a fully developed ability to shift from self-sensing to self-observation. As mentioned in Chapter 2, feelings are viral—pleasant or unpleasant—and get readily passed around through emotional contagions.[12] Ideally we want an emotional body that is free and has strong immunity. *This does not mean being apathetic, passive, cold, or hardened.* It does not mean being free of emotion. It means the emotional body is free to be self-determined. It is no longer reactive; its behavior is not dependent on outside influences, and it's not so susceptible to emotional contagions. A liberated emotional body is sensitive to inergy influences but does not morph into an obese body or shrink into an emaciated body by intense emotional input. Rather, it vibrates at high frequency, is compassionate, and is dynamically responsive to the moment. It is resilient: simultaneously strong and flexible. Immune strengthening demands a strong constitution and is not to be tried without proper emotional body hygiene and health treatments already in place.

The exercise[13] below begins with listening to soothing music. The emotional body is very sensitive to sound[14] to the extent that pharmaceutical music is available that has been shown to relieve certain emotional states and enhance others.[15] Choose music wisely. For this exercise, and in general, it's best to use music that is beautiful, uplifting, inspirational, and that has no lyrics, since lyrics can be a distraction. Avoid music that is hard driving, emotionally activating, or has any negative connotations for you. Music is like a drug for the emotional body so it's best to administer it carefully. Western Classical and New Age music are probably safe choices. In this exercise music is used as an anchoring influence, to help ground the emotional body. Once grounded, the exercise is unusual in that it asks you to visualize an emotionally upsetting scenario. The intent is to expose your emotional body to intensity and help it not to react unless you want it to.

Exercise: Immune Strengthening
Application: At least once a week, to train and free the emotional body. Only for use after basic hygiene and treatments have been in place and you are feeling emotionally healthy.
Supplies: Music player and beautiful, soothing music
Time: 4 minutes

- Find a place in which you can focus without distraction.

- Be in a seated position, as comfortable as possible.

- Take a couple of slow, deep breaths.

- Listen to beautiful music for at least 1 minute before proceeding to the next step. Keep the music running for the remainder of the exercise.

- Gently close your eyes and intentionally shift your attention away from an external focus toward an internal focus.

- Focus your intent on strengthening your emotional body to be more resilient and less susceptible to emotional contagions.

- When you are ready, begin to visualize two aggressive dogs fighting. See them viciously biting and tearing at each other. See the bleeding wounds. Use your intent to witness this scene with pure observation, remaining as emotionally neutral as possible throughout.

- Observe the scene for about 2 minutes. The intent of the exercise is to train the emotional body to observe the scene without getting emotionally activated.

- When about 2 minutes have passed, let go of the visualization. Focus on your breathing to help anchor your attention in real time. Take a couple of deep breaths. Feel your feet on the floor. Whenever you are ready open your eyes.

- Note the results of the exercise: For how long were you able to stay in pure observation mode without getting emotionally activated?

- In the case of emotional activation, use the treatments described in this chapter as needed to transform the inergies.

Immune Strengthening is an exercise. It's not meant to suggest that if you see two animals fighting you should stand by and watch, doing nothing. If this happens in life, the exercise is meant to enable you to choose a sensible response and not automatically jump into emotional reactivity. As a further immune strengthening exercise, apply this technique to watching emotionally intense movies or reading dramatic stories. The benefits of the exercise can carry over into many aspects of your life, giving you expanded choices and more freedom.

Compassion Container

Having covered the basics of immune strengthening, we are now ready to move into the important arena of protecting your immunity while directly interacting with other people's emotions. Because emotional inergies are highly contagious and emotional body neglect so prevalent, infectious emotions abound. This makes attending to the emotional needs of others a necessary home healthcare skill. Helping others can also strengthen your own emotional immune system by exposing you to emotional "germs" and building your immunity. The following exercise shows how to deal with emotional contagions in ways that help the other person while protecting your own emotional body health.

To continue with the physical body metaphor, say a loved one is slicing vegetables and accidentally suffers a cut. Most likely you would assist by getting a paper towel or band-aid and offering sympathy. Even when it comes to undesirable ailments, a loved one feeling nauseated, you would speak comforting words and fetch a bucket. But when a loved one is directing undesirable emotional inergy our way, sympathy and comfort are often scarce. It's common to fall into an awkward silence, at best, or, more likely, to get upset in response. We may say hurtful things or walk away, making the situation worse and abandoning our loved one in a time of need. When it comes to emotional upset it's hard to respond in a helpful way. Because emotions are so highly contagious, both emotional bodies get activated creating an Amplifier Loop. We are not able to help others if we are overtaken by our own emotional reactivity.

The following exercise[16] is a way to offer assistance when someone is upset with you. It consists of holding a compassion container for another person's emotional upset. The exercise is to be used to help the emotional body. *It is not meant to solve the problem or resolve the issue.* It is simply meant to attend to the needs of an upset emotional body. The exercise interrupts Amplifier Loops and helps the body to reset. After the emotional charge has dissipated, you may choose to go back and address the issue.

Holding a container means allowing the person to express their feelings while you remain fully present and non-reactive. You have enough emotional resilience to compassionately help the person in need. Holding a compassion container requires that you remain emotionally present in a positive way. It's not about closing down your emotional body or theirs; you stay present and supportive while they emote. You can only accomplish this if your emotional body is healthy. Otherwise your body will resonate with the heavy frequencies and morph into one of its unbalanced postures. It will want to go obese and take over, producing drama behavior, or go anorexic and disappear, producing android behavior. If this happens to you, the treatments described above are needed—Assurance, Tapping, or Reversal.

The compassion container is established through words and involves the mental body. It has two steps: repeating and validating. Start by repeating back what the person has said. The purpose of repeating is twofold. First, it gives you something to do. You are much less likely to become reactive if you have something to do. It also affirms that you are listening. Do your best to reflect back what was said as accurately as you can. For example, the upset person says, "*You are so critical. You think you are the expert on everything!*" Your response would be, "I'm being critical and acting like the expert on everything." This is not an admission of guilt, you are just letting the person know that you heard what they said. Repeating a derogatory statement about yourself may seem a stretch but can be mastered with practice.

The next step, validate, asks even more of you. It requires that you temporarily abandon your position and adopt the perspective of the upset person. It means affirming their experience. You want to express acceptance of their way of seeing things and verbally fill out the picture as best you can to show your understanding. Step inside the person's experience and speak from that viewpoint. Take their perspective and give it your voice; standing inside their shoes for a moment. Saying, "I understand" is very helpful in supporting the person's viewpoint. Those two words can go a long way.

With a healthy emotional body you can validate relatively easily. However, it may not feel good at first. You likely will find yourself validating untruths about yourself. The exercise requires that you repeat back what was said at the expense of your own self-defense and point of view. Dropping your way of seeing things is only temporary, though, for the duration of the exercise, or as long as it takes for the person's emotional body to calm down. You can always go back to your viewpoint after that; don't worry, it will still be there! You don't lose anything by temporarily abandoning your perspective and adopting another's. Instead, you gain. Your world becomes bigger because you are able to see things from the other person's point of view in addition to your own. You expand your awareness. Here are some examples of what validation might sound like in emotionally charged situations.

Example 1
Person: "You never listen to me!"
You: "It seems like I don't listen to you and I can understand that because when things get heated I interrupt and talk over you and you don't get a chance to finish."

Example 2
Person: "You always stick up for her!"
You: "You're saying I always stick up for your sister. I can understand that because I tell you to leave her alone and ask you to apologize to her, so it seems like I am always taking her side."

Example 3
Person: You lied! You said you would finish that project by Thursday and you didn't!
You: "I lied because I said I would finish the project by Thursday and I didn't. I can understand that because you were counting on me and I let you down."

If after validating the person's experience the upset continues, you can try two more simple techniques. You can offer an apology and/or ask the person what you can do to make the situation right. An apology is similar to the ointment of assurance; it is very soothing to the emotional body. An apology is not an admission of guilt or wrongdoing. It simply means you are sorry, as in sorrowful. In other words, you are sad. It's likely you would feel sad when someone you care about is upset and there is no harm in saying so. In fact, it's helpful. It soothes an upset emotional body. In addition, just like asking a person with an upset stomach what they need, you can ask an emotionally upset person what they need and do your best to offer that. Hopefully they can tell you and there is no harm in asking.

Exercise: Compassion Container
Application: As needed, when someone you are interacting with is emotionally upset with you
Time: Varies, depending on the situation

- When someone is upset, remain emotionally present and compassionate.

- Repeat what was said with care and an attitude of compassion.

- Validate the person's experience, even at the expense of your own.

- If the upset continues, apologize and/or ask the person what you can do to make things better, and do it.

From basic hygiene to immune strengthening and advanced techniques, a healthy emotional body is vital to your overall wellbeing. There are countless opportunities to use the exercises described for optimal emotional body health and fitness. However, the emotional body not only responds to emotional inergies, it is also highly influenced by its neighbor, the mental body. The next step is to look into the functioning of your mental body.

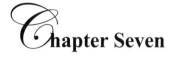

Chapter Seven

Your Mental Body

In a remote location in rural Wisconsin ten like-minded people gathered in the summer of 1999 to share their mutual interest in exploring the unusual. During one interactive session the ten stood in a room with metal forks in their hands while being instructed to bend the forks with their minds. The facilitator, Jack Houck,[1] was a retired aeronautical engineer who had worked for Boeing for 42 years. Jack had also met with Hal Puthoff and Russell Targ at the Stanford Research Institute during the government-sponsored experiments investigating parapsychological phenomena.[2] The purpose of the CIA-initiated research was to determine if psychic phenomena, such as remote viewing, would have utility for intelligence collection. The results of the investigations were so compelling that the project spanned over 20 years.

Inspired by Puthoff and Targ, Jack went on to develop his own research program, and his psychic abilities as well. He had spent decades hosting psychokinesis gatherings, successfully training thousands of participants to use their minds for remote viewing and metal bending. With Jack's guidance, Wisconsin participants stared at their respective forks, simultaneously focusing their will upon them, intending their chosen fork to bend while repeatedly shouting, "Bend! Bend! Bend!" Nothing happened. Nervous laughter filled the room. Everyone felt silly. Jack coached the participants to redouble their efforts. *Hold the focus. Use your mind to connect with the fork. Intend. Command the fork to bend! Then let go! Let go!* Participants obliged. Suddenly, as if on cue, the forks simultaneously turned to rubber and could be molded like taffy into twisted shapes. I was one of the participants. I still have my convoluted fork.

As we continue to explore the human energy constitution, moving up the inergy (energy/information) continuum from the emotional body, the next higher frequency band contains the mental body. Because the mental body is vibrating at quite a fast speed, it has particular potency. The mental body is responsible for processing inergies on the mental plane. It occupies the frequency range in between your emotional and universal bodies. Because of this, the mental body is highly influenced both by emotions and by universal inergies.

The two-way process between the mental and emotional bodies is most noticeable. When you are emotionally distressed, thinking easily becomes impaired. You may find that your mind gets foggy and confused, making it hard to focus, or that your thoughts become influenced by lower frequency emotional inergies. Amplifier Loops can also occur: if your emotional body is triggered into heavy feelings, your mental body can begin to vibrate at a resonant frequency. The low frequency thoughts, in turn, influence your emotional body and heavy feelings get reinforced, creating a self-perpetuating loop. Just as feelings are food for the emotional body, thoughts are the substance of the mental body.

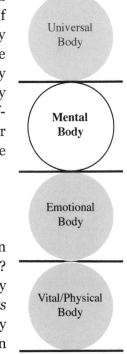

Thoughts Are Things

What if you could see thoughts, your own and those of others. What would they look like? How would they move? What impact would they have? From the perspective of inergy, *thoughts are things*. We cannot see them but inergetically they have size, shape, and they behave in certain predictable ways. Because they occupy the mental frequency range of your inergy constitution, thoughts vibrate at a high frequency. This gives them great potency. Your thoughts have the capacity to create action at a distance and to impact your own emotional and mental bodies as well. In fact, your thoughts are probably the most important factor in determining your overall health.

To have a healthy mental body you need to have healthy thoughts. But what determines the health factor of a thought? To understand this we need to look into how thoughts work by studying their effects. Luckily, the effects of thoughts have been well documented in hundreds of controlled experiments.[3] Thought has been shown to impact a variety of living things such as people, animals, insects, plants and cells. It has also been proven to impact inanimate objects such as chocolate, water, and electronic devices, including computers. Distance, from a few feet to thousands of miles, doesn't limit the effects. If there were ever any doubt that thoughts are things, recent research shows that thoughts can actually be stored and transported, just like little passengers, when they are attached to an electronic device.

One of my favorite studies from Stanford University demonstrates many of the incredible qualities that thoughts possess in one experiment. It involves something called an Intention Imprinted Electronic Device (IIED), or host device, for short.[4] This is a simple electronic object, about the size of a household remote control, that has been used to store thought so it can be isolated and transported to different locations to study its effects. The thoughts stored in host devices come from carefully selected individuals who have developed their mental bodies so they are able to produce clear and potent thoughts. Usually they are long time meditators who have mastered the power of concentration. They sit in a quiet room and purposefully focus their intent on the requested outcome and direct those thoughts into the host device.

In one experiment, an intention-host device was imprinted with the specific thought to change the pH of water by one unit. Anyone who owns a swimming pool knows that pH levels do not quickly change on their own without some kind of chemical intervention. The pH host device was then shipped to a location 2000 miles away along with others (the control devices) that were not imprinted. This was done to make sure none of the researchers on the receiving end knew which device was imprinted so their bias wouldn't affect the outcome of the experiment.

The results were clear. Only when the host device was put near a container of water did the water show the intended pH change. What was not expected, but also happened, was that water containers within 150 feet of the intention-infused device began to show changes as well.[5] Host devices have also been used by scientists to show how thought can significantly alter the development of fruit fly larvae and the activity of liver enzymes, among other things. By isolating intent through the host device and sending it to a different location these experiments help verify that human thought, and no other influence, is what makes the difference.

It's difficult to grasp that your private, personal thoughts could have such far-reaching effects. But the impact of thought is not reserved for trained meditators in controlled experiments; it is actually quite commonplace. Sometimes thoughts can be felt, like when someone is staring at you from behind and you sense it. Or when a loved one is sick and you pray for quick healing or send positive thoughts and the person gets better right away. There is also the familiar experience of the phone ringing and you know who is calling before you answer because you were just thinking of that person for no apparent reason. Most of us have experienced some kind of premonition, intuition, or mind-reading ability firsthand. If not, we know someone who has. Television shows featuring animal intuitives, psychics, or remote viewing have become mainstream. But how do these kinds of things happen?

We have been taught to believe that psychic experiences are meaningless, coincidental, or are exclusive to people with special powers. However, recent studies and new ways of evaluating prior research show that psychic experiences are very real and happen frequently, having been verified by literally thousands of scientific experiments conducted over the years.[6] Psychic experiences are not isolated or coincidental; they are common and predictable. So common, in fact, that the Institute of Biosensory Psychology boasts a 100% success rate in teaching people telekinesis (moving objects without touching them) while holding the Guinness record for teaching the most people in the shortest time.[7] Psychic experiences happen because of the capability of the mental body and the nature of thought, not because someone is highly evolved or more spiritual. Just as being a good dancer doesn't mean a person is spiritually adept, having psychic capacities doesn't either. If you have a mental body you can be psychic. In other words, we are all psychic to varying degrees.

Thought-Forms

Since thoughts greatly impact your inergy health, the first step to having a healthy mental body requires learning about thoughts and their qualities. Most of us cannot see thoughts, and, in fact, many psychics lack this capacity as well; they are primarily attuned to the emotional realm. So we must turn to those who are more advanced to learn how thoughts behave. The following information comes from a team of adept clairvoyants who could see thoughts. They dedicated their talents to research, meticulously describing and cataloging what they saw so the rest of us could understand thoughts better.[8] The clairvoyant team was observing thoughts that had been discharged into the atmosphere (no longer solely inside a person's inergy field), therefore they used the term *thought-form* to make this distinction. Let's look into the life of a typical thought-form.

Much like people, thought-forms come in different shapes, colors, and sizes (see Figure 7.2). The shape and size of a thought-form depend on its content, which is determined by your mental body; the color is determined by your emotional body. Thoughts are constantly in motion for as long as they exist and each individual thought-form moves at a certain speed. If you could see a thought it

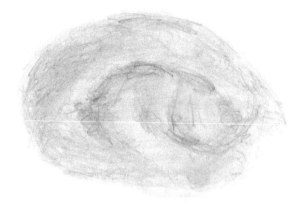

Figure 7.2 Artist's depiction of a typical thought-form. The fuzzy edges indicate the thought is somewhat unclear, while the dark areas inside show lower frequency emotional content. (Inspired by the work of Annie Besant and C.W. Leadbeater, *Thought-Forms,* Wheaton, Ill: Quest, 1986. Illustration by Bob Pedersen. Used with permission.)

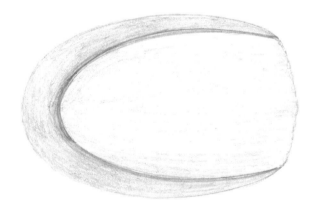

Figure 7.3 Artist's depiction of a coherent thought-form. The well-defined edges indicate the thought is clear. The light and uniform interior shows higher frequency emotional content. (Inspired by the work of Annie Besant and C.W. Leadbeater, *Thought-Forms,* Wheaton, Ill: Quest, 1986. Illustration by Bob Pedersen. Used with permission.)

would look like a fuzzy colored image floating through water.[9] From the floating thought-form a vibration radiates out. The color and vibrational rate of the thought are determined by your emotional body. Your emotions literally color your thoughts. The brilliance and depth of color indicate the strength and activity of your feelings. Low frequency emotions slow down the vibrational rate of the thought-form whereas higher frequency emotions speed it up.

In general, a healthy mental body is able to hold a focus and has the power of concentration. An unhealthy mental body is unable to hold a focus, lacks the power of concentration, and is overly susceptible to the emotional body (which often is unhealthy as well). Essentially, a healthy mental body produces clear, coherent thought-forms. However, I don't mean thought-forms that are logical or comprehensible. Instead, I am using the word *coherent* in the physics sense, as it is used to describe the make-up of light. Lasers, for example, produce coherent light that travels far and is very potent and clean. This is in contrast to the diffuse, weak light produced by a household lightbulb.

A clear thought-form has substance that is consistent and unified within itself. The content of the thought-form is uniformly vibrating at the same frequency. Clear thought-forms are characterized by having aerodynamic shapes and well-defined, distinct borders (see Figure 7.3). The clarity of a thought determines the definiteness of its outline. The clearer the thought, the more streamlined it is and the further it can travel. If your mental body is healthy, clear, and possesses the power of concentration you can produce coherent thought-forms. Like laser beams, these thought-forms travel at high speed and often reach their targets. On the other hand, if your mental body is weak, unhealthy, or unable to hold a focus, it will produce thought-forms that are fuzzy, slow, and unlikely to reach their destination.

The condition of your mental body also determines the lifespan of a thought. The distance, force and persistency of a thought depend on the strength and clarity of the original thought. In fact, clarity of thought is the most important factor in determining the distance a thought-form can travel, as well as its staying power. That's why research on intent, such as the study above with the host-devices, is usually done using trained meditators. Most bona fide forms of meditation involve calming your emotional body, clearing your mental body of extraneous thoughts, and holding a focus, thereby improving your power of concentration. Consistent meditation practice such as this often results in a fit, healthy mental body capable of producing potent, coherent thought-forms. Since the condition of your mental body is a large determinant in your overall health, this explains why meditation has so many proven health benefits affecting the vital/physical, emotional, mental, and universal bodies.

Types of Thought-Forms

In general, there are three types of thought-forms: 1) those that take on forms of their own; 2) those that resemble some physical form; and 3) those that resemble the image of the person who produced them. The first and most common type of thought is formed entirely out of emotional and mental inergies. These thought-forms take on shapes of their own, expressing their inherent qualities through the inergies they attract around them. They are like inergy magnets, attracting similar vibrations as they travel, and morphing into various shapes accordingly. They are conglomerations that contain multiple thoughts and thoughts mixed with feelings. This happens because most of our thoughts are not coherent. They are not pure, which compromises their potency and lifespan. Thought-forms act as magnets, attracting similar thoughts to them and growing larger in the process. You can see how important it is to pay attention to what you think, as your thoughts couple with other thoughts, amass together, and create enormous collective thought-forms.

The second type, thoughts that take on the replica image of physical forms, consist of thoughts you think about people or things that are familiar to you. These thoughts are formed out of your impressions of the actual physical appearance of the person or object. If you think of a friend or a house, thought-forms that resemble the friend or house hover around you. They appear as portraits of your friend or landscapes of the house. If you think of a painting you want to create, your ideas hover around you as little thought-form "pictures" and you utilize them in your creative process.

Thought-forms that take on the image of the thinker happen when you think about yourself. Such thoughts may hover around you or travel great distances. If, for example, you are planning a vacation to a nearby resort and you picture yourself lounging at the pool, soaking up the sun, a thought-form of you can appear poolside at the resort. At first it may be very small in size but the more you think about yourself at the pool, the more inergy you add to it and the thought-form may eventually become life-sized, attracting corresponding inergies like a magnet. This explains why visualization and imagery are such powerful tools. However, the same is true for unpleasant thoughts. If you are afraid you'll end up in a bad hotel and you keep worrying about that, imagining yourself there, a thought-form of you can appear in a bad hotel. The more you think that worrisome thought, the larger the thought-form grows. Again, it's important to pay attention to what you think.

Thought-forms act as magnets.

If you think critically about yourself, those thought-forms hover around you and can produce undesirable side effects. Let's say you make a mistake and instead of letting it go you become self-critical. Since thoughts are magnetic, a variety of critical thoughts stream in. Eventually you change your focus and get busy with other things. You're able to stop the negative self-talk and have a decent day. But then at night when you're lying in bed, just before you fall asleep, seemingly out of nowhere, derogatory thoughts descend upon you. You can't sleep because you can't shut your mind off. This happens because your self-critical thought-forms from earlier can hover around you for a long time. While you're busy focusing on other things they are kept at bay but when a passive moment happens, they come back into your mind because they are still within the frequency range of your inergy field.

Thought-Form Behaviors

Your mental body produces thought-forms about yourself, about others, and about no one in particular. If a thought-form is directed at no one, it floats detached in the atmosphere broadcasting inergy vibrations similar to its own. If it doesn't contact a compatible mental body nearby, it disintegrates over time. If it succeeds in awakening a resonant vibration in the mental body of a nearby person, it gets absorbed by the person and reproduces the same thought. Therefore, by intentionally thinking positive thoughts, sending forth inspirational thought-forms, you can do great service to assist others.

If your thoughts or feelings are directed to a particular person, the thought-form moves toward the intended person and discharges itself in the mental and emotional bodies of that person. For example, if you send a thought of love strongly directed toward a particular person, it creates a thought-form that potentially travels to the person and remains in their inergy field as an agent of love. Whether or not the thought-form reaches its recipient depends on the condition of your mental body, primarily determined by your ability to focus and concentrate, as well as the health of your emotional body.

The idea of sending and receiving positive thought-forms may be very appealing, but what happens with negative thoughts? Do they hover around and do harm? Is there really something to the so-called evil eye? For a negative thought to have impact it must find inergies that are resonant with its low frequency vibration in the recipient's field. In other words, *you cannot be affected by the negative thoughts of others unless you already have similar negative thoughts in your inergy field*. The temptation has been to accuse others of "contaminating" us with negative energy. We hear a lot about "toxic" people or "bad vibes," but we must take responsibility for our own negative thoughts, which radiate out and magnetize resonant negative thoughts.

The same is true with negative emotions. If you react to a situation by getting angry, your emotional body becomes agitated and the vibrational rate of the body changes to that of anger. This usually passes in a few seconds but the more you indulge in anger, the more the overall "tone" of your emotional body is permanently affected. It becomes easier to give in to anger again because your emotional body gets conditioned to vibrating at that particular rate. This is the inergetic mechanism behind repetitive emotions and why the emotional body is so prone to addiction.

But what happens to negative thought-forms that do not find sympathetic inergies in their targets? Do they just keep traveling around like door-to-door salesmen until they find agreeable recipients? We already know that thought-forms directed at no one disintegrate if they don't contact a corresponding mental body nearby. But if a thought is directed at a particular person and cannot find a resonant vibration, interestingly enough, the thought rebounds from the recipient's field with proportional force, much like a boomerang, and returns to the sender. If you think negatively about someone and the thought-form is not resonant with that person, it will come back to you with equal force. Similarly, if someone thinks negatively about you, and if you have no resonant frequencies, their thought will rebound. Therefore, *the best protection is not to have negative thoughts in your field to begin with*. Then negative thought-forms have nothing to connect with.

We cannot be affected by low frequency inergies unless we already possess them. If there is no low frequency inergy for negative thoughts or feelings to adhere to, they will pass through you like water through a sieve. Thus, the best practice for mental body health is maintaining high frequency thoughts. These will construct a refined mental body that cannot respond to the vibrations of slower and denser inergies. The practice of attuning to high frequency thought-forms may sound a lot like denial (i.e., pretending the negative thoughts aren't there and only paying attention to the positive), but it is categorically different. Denial is a defense mechanism in which a painful reality is not allowed into conscious awareness. By definition, denial requires a lack of awareness whereas attuning to high frequency thought-forms is done with conscious awareness and free choice (more about this in Chapter 9). Just like you would choose fresh food over spoiled food, it's best to choose high frequency thought-forms.

Your Brain is an Antenna

It appears that your brain doesn't so much produce thoughts as it receives and transmits them. That's why scientists probing inside the human brain have been unable to find the mechanisms to account for memory, thought-formation, or consciousness. Thoughts exist in a realm that is outside of physical reality, outside of the physical brain, outside of the conventional dimensions of length, width, height, or even time.[10] The thought-form level of reality functions in the empty space between the particles that make up normal atoms and molecules.[11] That's why it's invisible to most of us and to typical measurement instruments. Your brain is an organ of receptivity and transmission. Your mental body, or mind, is the link between your physical brain and the thought dimension, between physical reality and thought reality.

Because your mental body produces thought-forms and your physical brain transmits and receives them, the quality of your thoughts is largely dependent upon what you are attuning your brain to receive. Similar to the receiver that's part of a home stereo system, you can use your brain to tune into whatever thought-forms you want. Just as radio stations offer a variety of music and information, a vast supply of thought-forms are readily available. If you don't like the programming, you can change the station. If your thoughts offend you, you can tune into something else. The choice is yours.

Signal Scramble

The mental and emotional bodies occupy distinct frequency bands, yet they heavily influence each other. The emotional body is a lower frequency range than the mental, making emotional inergy denser so it more easily affects the refined inergies of the mental body. Compare a computer chip with a household fuse box. Like a computer chip, the mental body has refined circuitry with greater capabilities whereas the fuse box is like the emotional body, strong voltage and more raw power. Problems can occur when a highly charged emotional body causes interference with the mental.

A particular type of interference, and the most difficult to deal with, happens when your mental body's signals get scrambled by incoming emotional inergies and deliver a distorted picture of reality while you are unaware this is happening. It's like an electrical arc-flash that can occur in power systems and electronic equipment. Electrical current can jump from one conductor to another through a normally nonconductive medium. This results in extreme high temperatures capable of frying circuits or vaporizing most materials. When controlled, these arcs can be used positively, such as in melting metals in welding. If uncontrolled, they can wreak havoc.

In the case of your emotional and mental bodies, inergy can arc from your activated emotional body to your mental body and cause mental signals to get scrambled. When this happens your thought process becomes temporarily distorted but you don't know it. You can inaccurately perceive and misinterpret reality. Your mental body delivers a distorted picture but, because you perceive via your mental body, you can't see that the picture is distorted. You can make things up, create fantasy stories in your head, and yet be completely unaware that you are doing so. For the duration of the signal scramble, the make believe story becomes your reality.

In electrical systems, repeated energy arcs can eventually fry circuitry. An extreme high voltage arc-flash can damage the lower voltage power supply. In the case of your inergy bodies, the mental body is lower voltage than the emotional. It is higher up on the inergy continuum, meaning, it contains high frequency, refined inergies and less raw voltage. Your mental body is filled with delicate circuitry. Long-term arcing or intense arc-flashes produce severe signal distortion that can translate into dementia[12] or other mental health issues. Although this is relatively rare, short-term and mild signal scrambles are quite commonplace. You've probably experienced them many times. There are two clues that a signal scramble is happening: 1) your reaction is disproportionate to the situation at hand, and; 2) your reaction is predictable. Let's look at an example.

Todd's father, Harry, was angry and controlling. He ruled his family with an iron fist and, consequently, Todd spent his entire childhood in fear of his father's wrath. Always suspicious and mistrusting, one of Harry's favorite tactics was to relentlessly interrogate young Todd. Todd found his father's large frame and booming voice so intimidating that he would look away in fear, unable to answer his father's questions. This infuriated Harry who would angrily demand that Todd look him in the eye. The anxiety-filled child would force himself to look, only to be met with dagger eyes staring him down. Soon after, a painful spanking would follow.

Fast forward to the present when Todd is in an intimate relationship with Heather. Like any couple, they have their difficulties. But their relationship is a good one, healthy and stable for the most part. Heather probably looks at Todd a million times a day, often staring lovingly into his eyes, and he welcomes her gaze. However, when they are having the occasional heated argument a strange thing happens. They will exchange angry words followed by a tense silence. During that silence, if Heather is looking into his eyes anticipating his next words, Todd grows visibly agitated. Eventually he explodes, demands that she stop staring him down, and storms out of the room. The stunned Heather scratches her head and wonders what on earth is going on.

Todd is experiencing a signal scramble: his reaction is disproportionate and predictable. During the heat of the argument, his emotional body gets activated into anxiety. As the intensity increases, the spike in emotional inergy causes a "power surge" that arcs to his mental body. There, the influx of high voltage "foreign" inergy scrambles his mental body and distorts his perception. Instead of seeing Heather for who she is, completely unbeknownst to Todd, he mistakes her for his volatile, aggressive father and reacts accordingly. None of this is conscious or intentional.

There is a way out of the signal scramble and it requires the ability to observe your thoughts and emotions instead of being pulled into them and becoming reactive. For this we need another kind of mental capacity. We need to use our "second brain."

Two Minds in One

Your mental body actually has two aspects that function differently, a higher and lower mental capacity. It's like having two minds in one. The higher mind is more inclusive in its orientation while the lower mind has a narrower focus. Your lower mind is designed to process intellectual information and is referred to as the *concrete mind*. This mind is primarily externally focused. It concerns itself with the day-to-day functioning of ordinary life. It is responsible for facts, logical reasoning, and analysis. Your concrete mind gives you the capacity for rational thought. It allows you to judge and make distinctions. It is the storehouse for facts and acquired knowledge. It is also the seat of common sense. Worry belongs to the concrete mind, as do the mundane thoughts that often digress into noisy mental chatter. The concrete mind is the predominant mental aspect for most people.

Your higher mind is not so concerned with concrete information. Called the *conceptual mind*, it is designed to process abstract principles, generalized patterns, and concepts. Thoughts connected with the conceptual mind are qualitatively different than those of the concrete mind. Your conceptual mind is responsible for understanding, insights, and truth. Unlike the concrete mind that functions to separate and distinguish, thoughts from your conceptual mind are inclusive in nature.

This mind has the capacity to observe a situation and get a broad overview, to go to a higher level and identify patterns. It is very good at formulating theories and seeing trends. For this reason, the conceptual mind is designed to produce those "ah-ha" experiences when you are able to connect the dots and gain insight into a situation or problem. Usually the newfound insight completely shifts your perspective, resulting in a deeper understanding.

Higher and lower mental capacities are not to be confused with left/right brain functioning. Since the right brain is associated with a softer focus and the left is considered the detail brain, there is a tendency to equate the right brain with higher mental functioning and the left with lower. But this is not accurate. Both brain hemispheres are involved in higher and lower mental functioning. It's possible to have a soft focus (right brain) and still be functioning at the concrete level. It's also possible to be very detail-oriented (left brain) and be functioning in a higher mental capacity. The goal is to be whole-brained in whatever we do, to see the details within the broader perspective and to see the more expansive view as well as the details. The concrete and conceptual minds involve both brain hemispheres.

Director's Mode

Your conceptual mind possesses the power of observation. It allows you to step out of an experience and see it from a bigger perspective, to see how the situation came about. It allows you to witness a situation and to see behind things. When you watch a movie on DVD, for example, you typically have the option to play the movie or to watch any number of behind-the-scenes features, such as the Director's Notes. If you play the movie, the story unfolds with all of its drama. If you watch the Director's Notes you go behind-the-scenes to see how the movie was made. You get background information and insights about the characters. Then when you watch the movie you have a broader perspective—you can see the action packed drama and know what went into the making of it.

In real life there is a huge difference between being *in* a problem versus being able to *observe* the problem. When you are in a problem, you are an actor in the movie. You are in the drama. The intensity is high, events loom larger than life, and your concrete brain is calculating all of the variables trying to figure out what to do. In contrast, when you observe the problem from the Director's chair, you shift into conceptual thinking and are able to rise above the situation. You can see it from a different angle, as if you were directing the movie instead of starring in it. By observing the problem you are able to view the story as it unfolds plus you also get the information from behind-the-scenes. You are in a better position to call the shots because you witness the action instead of being in it. Perspective is gained. By using Director's Mode, your understanding of the problem is broadened and expanded. It includes the behavior of the characters and the dramatic storyline while allowing you access to information about the characters' motivations, the larger context, and the background stories—including yours. When using your conceptual mind and observing the problem from Director's Mode your world is expanded.

> There's a big difference between being *in* a problem versus *observing* the problem.

In the story of Todd and Heather earlier in this chapter, if Todd had switched into Director's Mode to understand the conflict with Heather, he could have broadened his perspective, observed the situation, and perhaps not reacted so strongly. Afterward, he could have gone "behind-the-scenes" to see that his reaction was disproportionate to the situation, a big clue that a signal scramble had happened. In following this clue, he could potentially see that Heather's staring at him was the spark that triggered the scramble. He could then trace that trigger back to his father and bring awareness to his automatic reaction. Sharing this insight with Heather could help prevent repeat occurrences.

Let's look at another example. Brooke had gotten herself into a tough financial situation. She was living way beyond her means and had all of her credit cards maxed out to the tune of $23,000. Her only safety net was that she had bought some gold back in 1999 when the price was $340/oz. She was holding out, trying not to sell it because it was all she had. When she first bought the gold she promised herself she would keep it until it hit $800/oz. In November of 2007, gold climbed from $740 to $842. Right at the same time Brooke hit her debt limit and had to pay off at least one of her credit cards by November 15th. She had exhausted all other options. For the funds to clear her account, she had to either sell her gold on Friday, November 9th, or wait until the following Monday. Her clear intuitive sense was to sell on Friday.

Friday morning arrived and she got up early to check the price and sell the gold. It was $832 an ounce and still climbing. She was ecstatic. She went to the website of her gold holding and logged into her account where an article popped up about gold and its future. The article was very optimistic. She then thought to search around and read a few other articles to gain perspective. As usual, the experts' opinions were mixed. Some were predicting a sell-off while others were saying the precious metal was only beginning to rally. Which would it be? Gold had climbed substantially over the past few days, but would it continue in that direction for the next two days? Should she wait to sell on Monday? She decided to read more.

She studied the trends, looked at the graphs, and weighed the pros and cons. She poured over several articles and charted the results. Their analysis, along with her own conclusions, told her to stay in for two more days. She decided not to sell, confident gold would climb even further by Monday. At worst she calculated it may drop a few dollars, according to recent trends, but it was well worth the risk because the chances were far better it would increase. She desperately needed every cent she could get and hoped to sell for maximum profit.

On Monday morning Brooke logged on to her gold account, anxious to see how much further the precious metal had climbed and ready to press the sell key. When the website popped up, gold had dropped an astounding $52 an ounce, from $842 to $790. Brooke was devastated. *What happened? Why were the majority of experts so off base? Why did she listen to them anyway? What could she do?* She was miserable and felt like a victim. After a period of blaming others she realized that, looking back, her intuitive sense had been to sell the gold on Friday and not wait. It was loud and clear, she simply overrode it. This prompted a round of self-blame. *Why didn't she listen to her intuition? Why did she override it? When will she ever learn?* She was even more miserable, blaming herself because she should have known better.

When she felt herself spiraling downward, Brooke knew she'd better do something to intervene. She didn't want to suppress her feelings and force herself to focus on something happy, hoping the distressing feelings would go away. She also didn't want to wallow in misery much longer. She remembered a friend saying, "No experience is ever wasted. Every experience has a purpose and the purpose is to grow and become better." Brooke asked herself, *What am I supposed to learn from this? That I am stupid and mess everything up? That I blew it?*

Then she took her friend's advice more seriously and began to look at the situation in earnest, trying to discover how she could grow and become a better person from it. She realized that becoming better meant she had to stop the self-criticism (the two are mutually exclusive). She discovered that she could either deride herself for not selling at the right time or she could pay attention to the fact that her intuition was absolutely clear, strong, and correct. She decided to appreciate the accuracy of her intuition. She congratulated herself on getting this insight.

But then self-criticism returned. *Why couldn't I have gotten this insight and still sold the gold at the higher price? Why did I have to miss that opportunity to get this learning?* She probed deeper and discovered that if she had followed her intuition and sold the gold on Friday, the potency of her intuition would have easily been lost to the triumph of her success. She probably would have written it off as luck and quickly moved on. Or, worse, she would have been gloating so much she would have missed it altogether. The loss of the money is what caused her to stop and reflect on the situation. To put it another way, she needed to lose the money in order to really notice the clarity and accuracy of her intuition. When Brooke got this insight she experienced an immediate internal shift. She was able to calm down and let go of thinking about the situation. More importantly, she was able to stop blaming herself and others. She felt free, even grateful for the situation.

Internal experiences like these are difficult to describe in words because invariably they end up lacking. They sound overly simplistic, at best, or silly, at worst. The experience is so subjective, subtle, and specific to the individual and situation that reading about it can leave you with many unanswered questions. Perhaps you've had experiences similar to Brooke's so you can fill in the missing pieces and make sense of what I am describing. I hope you have the "referential hooks" to hang this information on.

In Brooke's story, she was engaging her concrete mind when she was analyzing the gold market and its future. She was strategizing, calculating and trying to decide what to do. She was still utilizing her concrete mind when she missed the mark and was trying to figure out where she went wrong. Her concrete mind continued to engage when she was stuck in blame. Then something shifted. She began to engage her conceptual mind when she stepped back and started to look at the situation from a broader viewpoint. Her conceptual mind allowed her to observe her own behavior in a neutral way, without emotionality or the negative judgment of her concrete mind. She was able to shift out of blame and broaden her perspective to see things that were previously invisible. She took the

Director's chair, went behind-the-scenes and got insights into her own behavior.

Will this bring back the money she lost by waiting to sell her gold? No. Will it help her pay off her credit card debt? Maybe. From the perspective of inergy, Brooke recalibrated her entire system and is now magnetizing and radiating higher frequency inergies. She was also much more vitalized by the insight she gained than she was by being miserable, blaming herself and others. That vitality can help her solve the problem more effectively. Also, the new awareness to trust her intuition is a valuable resource for her future. She can use her intuition to help solve the cash flow problem in creative ways that otherwise may not have been available to her.

Ideally, we want to use both minds together, the concrete and the conceptual. Life necessitates that we process information at the concrete level and that we are able to go beyond that to a deeper, more expansive understanding of life events, of others, and of ourselves. Understanding often brings peace of mind and fulfillment, two high frequency conditions. To help come closer to maximizing our mental capacities, both concrete and conceptual, we must discover how to care for our mental body to help it be as healthy as possible.

Chapter Eight

Steps to a Healthy Mental Body

In general, there are seven mental body types and each one is prone to a certain set of behaviors with accompanying strengths and weaknesses.[1] Each mental body, regardless of type, has the potential for concentration and intelligence. Knowing your body type does not determine the extent to which you are utilizing your mental capacities. Instead, the body types describe how mental inergy is utilized when a body is healthy versus unhealthy.

Let's try to determine your mental body type. The following checklist contains statements about how you might think. This is not an IQ or intelligence test. It requires that you have some awareness about your thinking process. In other words, to think about how you think. Most of us are not accustomed to doing this. For the most part, we simply have a constant thought-stream running inside our heads without contemplating it. So, before beginning the checklist, engage your faculty of self-observation to witness your thought process as best you can. You may want to reflect on the workings of your mental body by referring back to the exercise from Chapter 2 in which you were asked to describe your mental body in words and to sketch it.

When you have a sense of how your mental body functions, complete the following checklist to discover your body type. The questions describe various ways of thinking. It's best to respond using your first impression without analyzing too much. There are no right or wrong answers. By answering as honestly as possible, you can discover more about your mental body.

Your Mental Body Type

Put an X next to each statement that applies to you.

_____   My mind is like a laser; I stay with one topic all the way through. (A)

_____   I can easily see another person's point of view. (B)

_____   When I think about a topic, my mind quickly branches off in many directions. (C)

_____   I tend to see both sides of an issue, no matter what the issue. (D)

_____   I love facts and remember many of them easily. (E)

_____   I am committed to a cause or principle and it shapes my thinking. (F)

_____   I like to do things in step-by-step order. (G)

_____   I have strong opinions about things and don't easily change my mind. (A)

_____   In an argument, I tend to soften. (B)

_____   My mind is quick, adaptable, and abstract. (C)

_____   I typically have a hard time making up my mind. (D)

_____   I easily follow the instruction manuals for home electronics and devices. (E)

_____   I have strong convictions about what I believe. (F)

_____   I enjoy making lists and checking things off. (G)

_____ I get straight to the point when talking to someone. (A)

_____ I don't like to debate, it makes me anxious. (B)

_____ I enjoy non-sequential, random processing. (C)

_____ In an argument I tend to compromise easily. (D)

_____ I love diagrams, maps, and models. (E)

_____ I focus on one thing at a time and see it through to completion. (F)

_____ I value efficiency and love to find shortcuts. (G)

_____ I easily see the essence of things and quickly "cut to the chase." (A)

_____ I ponder on things, see the whole, big picture, and take my time. (B)

_____ I love to brainstorm, jump around, and think outside the box. (C)

_____ I tend to feel more than think. (D)

_____ I need to research and analyze the facts in order to change my mind. (E)

_____ I have my chosen area of interest and that's what I am dedicated to. (F)

_____ I am good at organizing and creating systems. (G)

Scoring Your Results

Add up all your Xs and make a note of their corresponding letters.

Write your totals here:

_____ A _____ B _____ C _____ D

_____ E _____ F _____ G

Because there is overlap among the mental body types, you may rank high in more than one category.

- Most points in the A category - You tend to have a Direct mental body.

- Most points in the B category - You tend to have an Inclusive mental body.

- Most points in the C category - You tend to have a Web mental body.

- Most points in the D category - You tend to have a Fluid mental body.

- Most points in the E category - You tend to have a Detailed mental body.

- Most points in the F category - You tend to have a Dedicated mental body.

- Most points in the G category - You tend to have an Ordered mental body.

The Seven Body Types

There are seven mental body types. Each one has distinct qualities, strengths and weaknesses. When the mental body is healthy the strengths are most evident and when it is unhealthy the weaknesses are apt to take over. The seven types are:

- Direct
- Inclusive
- Web
- Fluid
- Detailed
- Dedicated
- Ordered

Direct Mind

The direct mind is one-pointed. It works like a laser beam, focusing on one thing at a time and steadfastly following it through to completion. If you have a direct mind, you see where you want to go and see the most linear route to get from here to there. You like to give advice and you don't waste words, which means you can come off as a know-it-all. Your mind works fast. You are able to cut through, grasp basic principles, and easily see the essence of things. You think straight to the point, never deviating from your course. This can make you seem a bit hard-headed, close minded or overly opinionated. You are prone to impatience, especially if you are dealing with someone who is not quite as direct as you.

Healthy: Laser-like focus, seeing the essentials, persistency, goal-oriented

Unhealthy: Hard-headed, opinionated, impatient, domineering

Inclusive Mind

This mind sees the whole big picture in complete detail. Encompassing everything can be an expansive task and for this reason the inclusive mental body can take some time to process information. The desire to embrace everything makes it hard to say no and can make you overly-sensitive. If you have this body type, you are contemplative and look for the global picture. You are prone to introspection, getting lost in your thoughts. You may come off as self-absorbed. You gravitate toward wisdom instead of facts and easily get pulled into your studies. Sometimes you study too much at the expense of taking action. Not only do you love to learn but also to teach. You have great respect for intuitive understanding.

Healthy: Seeing the whole, contemplation, wisdom, intuitive understanding

Unhealthy: Too much study, over-sensitivity, over-introspection, self-absorbed

Web Mind

A web mind, like the name suggests, branches out widely and quickly. If you have a web-like mental body, you will find that your mind is very fertile, filled with an array of ideas on abstract questions. You can adapt your thinking to anything. You love to brainstorm and are very good at it. A web mind is like the World Wide Web. When you visit a website, certain words are highlighted that provide links to related information. This is much like the web mind, quickly expanding into related issues and further abstractions. This penchant for big thinking can make you forget details. You are prone to becoming scattered, over-extended, and absent-minded. You may also use your creative and resourceful mind in manipulative ways.

Healthy: Wide views on abstract issues, brainstorming, mental fertility, adaptability

Unhealthy: Absent-mindedness, over-extension, manipulation, deviousness

Fluid Mind

If you frequently experience indecision, chances are you have a fluid mind. This mental body type is adept at seeing both sides of an issue. This makes you a great mediator because you can bridge opposing ideas and help people through conflict. You also have deep sympathetic understanding. But when your mind goes back and forth like a seesaw people may see you as moody or unstable. Because of your vacillating mind you often rely on your emotional body, especially when making decisions. You tend to do what feels comfortable and easy instead of doing what's right. You can be impulsive and over-reactive but your keen sensitivity also makes you highly perceptive.

Healthy: Sees both sides, sympathetic understanding, perceptive, intuitive

Unhealthy: Unstable, impulsive, over-reactive, moody, indecisive

Detailed Mind

The detailed mental body tends to carefully analyze and examine, not daydream or intuit. Thought is executed in a precise, linear, sequential manner. If you have this type of mental body you love facts and are able to memorize them easily and accurately. To change your mind you will need to have proof. You excel at critical thinking and may regard yourself as a skeptic, especially of the unseen world. This predisposes you to being critical and narrow-minded. You are fond of diagrams, maps, and models. You tend to be technically savvy, easily able to follow the user manuals for programming computerized devices and electronics. Your precise and systematic mind can make you a victim of over-analysis. You are also prone to being insensitive.

> Healthy: Precise thought, careful analysis, accuracy, technical ability

> Unhealthy: Over-analysis, narrow-mindedness, criticism, insensitivity

Dedicated Mind

The dedicated mental body is singularly devoted to a cause or principle that guides it. If you have a dedicated mind, you will have one area of interest that you are motivated by and passionate about. This acts as a filter that colors your thoughts accordingly, creating a monochrome effect. With one-pointed commitment, your unwavering devotion often makes you visionary in your chosen endeavor. Your enthusiasm is contagious, inspiring and influencing others to join in. The downside is that you are easily carried away by the cause. Your thinking can become narrow and rigid. Although you are refreshingly idealistic, you can become suspicious or intolerant of opposing ideas, prone to blind devotion.

> Healthy: Single-mindedness, dedication, enthusiasm, idealism

> Unhealthy: Narrow-mindedness, intolerance, rigidity, blind devotion

Ordered Mind

The ordered mind loves organization and efficiency. Thought process is carried out in a systematic way, step by step. You love to make lists and check things off. You possess a great capacity for self-discipline and perseverance, which makes you very organized, accurate, and detail-oriented. However, you can go overboard with this, get lost in details, and become finicky and fussy. You are very good at creating systems and economizing. You excel at following instructions and easily memorize things in sequential fashion. But if that sequence gets interrupted, it can be very distressing. Your natural organizational abilities and attention to detail border on perfectionism. Friends may accuse you of being too formal and encourage you to relax.

Healthy: Accuracy, organization, attention to detail, systematic

Unhealthy: Perfectionism, overly orderly, excessively organized, fussy

Knowing your mental body type is an important part of understanding your overall inergy constitution. Because of the high frequency range of the mental level, your mental aspect has a strong influence on your overall personality. Your mental body also plays a large role in your career, as, unlike the emotional body, it is a highly utilized resource in many occupations. The inergies of the mental level are vibrating at fast frequency and therefore have great influence on your other bodies.

This is most evident when we sleep and dream. Let's say you dream you are drowning, struggling to save your life. You are gasping for air and flailing in the water as the undertow pulls you down. Then suddenly you wake up and realize you were dreaming. You will find that your emotional body is filled with fear. On the physical level, your heart is racing and your breathing is rapid, as if you were actually drowning instead of lying in bed. However, the situation only happened in your mind. Because of the potency of its high frequency range, your mental body is like a control tower heavily directing your emotional and physical bodies to follow it.

Mental Body Hygiene

Now that you have a better understanding of your mental body type, let's take a look at a self-care program for the mental body. Following our format for the emotional body, the steps to a healthy mental body begin with basic hygiene practices to be done on a daily basis. However, after that the approaches differ. Because there is such emphasis placed on developing the mental body in schools and career training, the mental is not as neglected as the emotional body. Thus, it is not so much in need of care treatments. Instead, the mental body requires a workout program to achieve optimal functioning and maintain its health. The exercises described below are useful for all seven body types.

Healthy Head

Basic hygiene for this body begins with some awareness of your body type so you can pay attention to enacting the healthy qualities of your type and avoiding the unhealthy. This exercise constitutes an ongoing basic hygiene practice.

Exercise: Healthy Head
Application: To enact healthy functions for your mental body type.
Time: Ongoing

- Consult the checklist above to review your mental body type along with its healthy and unhealthy tendencies.

- Throughout the day, pay attention to your mental body and make healthy choices.

Mental Body Mirror Check

The basic hygiene program for the mental body includes examining the body through a mirror check. For hygienic reasons, it's important to assess your mental body each day so you can make minor adjustments before conditions get too extreme.

Exercise: Mental Body Mirror Check
Application: At least once a day, to assess the condition of your mental body
Time: 1-2 minutes

- Find a quiet place in which you can focus without distraction.

- Take a couple of slow, deep breaths. Close your eyes and intentionally shift your attention away from an external focus toward an internal focus, awakening your internal senses.

- Allow your physical body to relax.

- Allow your emotional body to relax.

- In your mind's eye, see a mirror in front of you. Instead of your physical body, this mirror is reflecting your mental body.

- Notice everything you can about your mental body. How does it look today? What color is it? Shape? Size? What stands out? Notice the details. Anything you need to adjust? Overall condition?

- Whenever this feels complete, open your eyes.

If your mental body is in need of assistance, use the exercises that follow to address the needs accordingly.

Intent-Setting

Thoughts are the substance of the mental body so keeping this body clean and healthy requires working directly with thought-forms on a daily basis through intent-setting. The exercise consists of engaging your conceptual mind, choosing a specific high frequency thought-form for your mental body to focus on, and utilizing the power of your intent to attract corresponding thought-forms. In this way it cleans the mental body and conditions it to vibrate at higher frequencies.

There are several factors to consider when selecting your intent-focus. In general, it's best to follow these guidelines:

- Be Positive

- Focus on You

- Keep Intent Simple

- Be in the Present

- Think Conceptual

Be Positive

When formulating your intention, it's common to focus on a problem. A typical intention may be to have less stress, to have the pain go away, or to stop being depressed. But these statements are focused on the very things you are trying to get rid of—stress, pain, and depression. Thoughts are like magnets. If you focus your mind on what you want to get rid of you are actually feeding inergy to those very things. Instead, focus on what you want to gain so you can magnetize inergies and be constructive. If you want to build a house, you need lumber and nails. Thought-forms are like lumber and nails—they build things. It's important to be very clear about what you want to build so you mobilize inergy toward manifesting what you want and stop feeding inergy to the problem.

It's also important to pay attention to the wording of your intent because words themselves are containers of thought-forms. The power of words has been verified by Dr. Masaru Emoto's work on the effects of intention on water.[2] At first, the water was infused with intent by adept meditators. But then simply applying word-labels to the water produced the same results. Labeling vials of water with typewritten words and then "freeze-drying" it showed how water gets imprinted with the information contained in the words. When the water is labeled with positive words such as *love* and *gratitude* beautiful, symmetrical, bright crystal patterns form. When the water is labeled with negative words like *hate* and *kill* the patterns are dark, ugly, and deformed. Words are containers of inergies and each word has a distinct inergy "signature."

Words vibrate at particular frequencies and are encoded with specific information. Be mindful of what you are introducing into your field: *to name it is to claim it*. You want inergy that is high frequency and positive. For instance, if you want to stop smoking or lose weight, the tendency would be to have an intent-focus that is just that—to stop smoking or lose weight. But these statements actually reinforce the message of "*smoking*" and "*weight*" in your inergy field because the intent-focus contains those very words. Inserting the word *stop* in front of the word *smoking* doesn't take away the particular thought-forms and inergies encoded in the word *smoking*.

If your tendency is to focus on a problem (overweight) or what you want to get rid of (smoking), ask yourself these questions: *"If I woke up tomorrow morning and this problem was completely resolved, never to return, what would that bring me? What would I have then that I don't have now? What quality do I want to awaken in myself to help me with this problem?"* These questions help point you in the direction of positive, high frequency intentions. You might find that if you stopped smoking, you would be free. Or if you lost weight, you would feel energized. Your intent-focus would then be: *"I am free,"* or *"I am energized."* You might find that discipline could help you so, *"I have discipline,"* would be your intent.

Focus on You

The second guiding principle for intent-setting is to focus on you. It's tempting to make intentions that involve others because so often it seems other people are the problem! This is especially true if you are struggling with a particular individual. Other-centered intentions sound like this: *"I want my boyfriend to be more caring. I want my boss to be generous and kind. I want to help my mom stop complaining all the time."* When the impulse arises to focus your thoughts on another person, ask yourself this question: *"What quality do I want to awaken in myself to help me deal with this person?"* Then make an intention that is focused on activating that particular quality in you.

For example, let's say you are struggling in a relationship and you believe your partner is insensitive to your needs. If you ask yourself what quality you can awaken in yourself to help you with the situation, you may realize that you need patience. That becomes your intent-focus. Or you may realize that you could be less demanding. Then, remembering that the best intentions are positive, you can find what "less demanding" might look like. It may take the form of being more accepting, allowing, or giving. Then your intent would become, *"I am accepting,"* or *"I allow,"* or

"*I am giving.*" In this way you are intentionally generating positive thought-forms about yourself that will hover in your inergy field and attract resonant positive thought-forms to you.

The question arises, will this serve to keep you in a bad relationship while ignoring the real problem? You can still address the insensitivity issue by talking with your partner. You can also choose to end the relationship. The exercise does not exclude these options. The benefits of intent-setting are two-fold. First, it helps to keep you from dwelling on the issue in your mind, a big waste of inergy. It also helps you to be constructive in your thinking and clean up your behaviors instead of automatically blaming your partner.

A second question arises about using your thoughts in a positive way to help someone. Can't you make a goal for your girlfriend to be more easy going? Or your sister to stop over-spending? When it comes to using intent to help others, the most potent effects are achieved—not from focusing on the outcome you want—but from intending the highest good for the person. Say your intent is for your sister to stop over-spending. She may not want to do that. You direct "stop spending" thought-forms to her and they resonate with her "spending" thought-forms and potentially reinforce the very thing you want to stop. If you focus your intent on "frugality," there is no resonant inergy in her field, therefore, the thought-form rebounds. However, if you reset your intention to focus on the highest good for your sister, there is likely some sympathetic inergy in her field for this thought-form to resonate with. It can go forth and activate similar thoughts in her that could potentially help her.

Similarly, if you want peace in the world, you can focus on achieving peace inside yourself. From the perspective of inergy, some of the most important social work you can do is to clean up your own mental body. Use your mental body to construct high frequency thought-forms. The problems of the world can seem overwhelming. However, keeping a clean mental body is something you can contribute. You are empowered to make a difference. The intent-setting exercise helps you do that by training your mental body to attune to high vibration thought-forms on a daily basis. In this way you can do your part and make a contribution to the greater good.

Keep Intent Simple

The next principle for intent-setting has to do with simplicity. If your intent becomes too wordy or contains many varied topics, the potency and focus of your intent becomes diffused. Rather than sending out a clear, concentrated thought-form, multiple forms are created, each one slightly weakened due to the sheer number. Rather than having a goal, "*I am free to breathe deep and easy and have abundant energy;*" instead try, "*I am free and energized.*" Think of your intent like a laser beam. Lasers are one-pointed. You want to be able to point the laser beam of your focused mind into the creation of a particular thought-form. When you do this, you attract corresponding thought-forms and infuse them with your inergy, thereby giving them potency. A positive Amplifier Loop is created that has great staying power.

Be in the Present

You want your intent-focus to be in the present tense, not future oriented. The biggest caveat to this is making goals that take place in the future. Often, we end up with an intent-focus that sounds something like this, "I *will be* more patient," or "I *want to be* more confident." To word your intention in this way means the completion of your goal happens at some point in the future, just out of your reach. Instead, you want to word the statement as if it already exists. Change it from an aspiration to a declaration. Change it from "I *will* be more patient," to "I *am* patient." From, "I *want to be* more confident," to "I *am* confident."

Think Conceptual

Finally, the best goals are conceptual. This means to devise an intent-focus that accesses the conceptual aspect of your mental body because thought-forms produced by your conceptual mind are vibrating at higher frequencies. It's tempting to make goals that address the concerns of the concrete mind but this may predispose you to lower frequency thought-forms.

A typical example would be an intention to have more money. This concrete mind thought-form will go forth and attract resonant thought-forms, of which there are many. It seems everyone wants more money and with varied motivations behind it. Some are motivated by greed, others by benevolence, still others by desperation. All of this emotional content colors the thought-form, making the desire for money a huge, conglomerate thought-form. Having this as your intent will contribute to growing and potentizing that collective thought-form. Is this really what you want?

Instead, ask yourself what having more money will do for you. Then you activate your conceptual mind. You might find that having more money can bring you joy, confidence, peace of mind, or creativity. Your intent then becomes, "*I am joyful, I have confidence, I have peace of mind,*" or "*I am creative.*" These conceptual mind thought-forms are vibrating at faster frequencies and are more pure. They are not conglomerate thought-forms. They have the potential to reach their target and effect positive change. Once you become resonant with joy, confidence, peace of mind and creativity, you will find it easier to make more money. Or you may realize that making more money is not so important after all; you are fulfilled in other ways. You also contribute to the collective joy and peace which helps reduce a global dependence on money for achieving such things.

The Intent-Setting exercise cleans your mental body by keeping it focused on what you want. It helps you utilize the power of your intent, engage your conceptual mind, and attune your mental body to high frequency thought-forms. This insures a clean and healthy body. The exercise is best done on a daily basis at the start of your day. Do your best to stay focused on your intention throughout the day. You can use reminders as needed (i.e., write yourself notes, put it on your calendar, put stickies on your mirror). If you want to check-in at the end of the day, you can review your intention to assess your success at manifesting it.

Exercise: Intent-Setting
Application: Best done once a day, upon starting your
day, to help the mental body stay attuned to higher
frequency inergies
Time: 1 minute

- Find a quiet place in which you can focus without
  distraction.

- Take a couple of slow, deep breaths. Close your eyes
  and intentionally shift your attention away from an
  external focus toward an internal focus, awakening
  your internal senses.

- Allow your physical body to relax.

- Allow your emotional body to relax.

- Ask yourself what you would like to focus on today.
  Remember the guidelines:
  - Be Positive
  - Focus on You
  - Keep Intent Simple
  - Be in the Present
  - Think Conceptual

- As clearly and purposefully as possible, send forth
  your intent so it may magnetize resonant inergies
  and manifest in your life.

- Whenever you are ready open your eyes.

- Do your best to remember your intention throughout
  the day (use reminders as needed).

- Review at the end of the day, if you'd like.

Once hygiene is in place, you can move on to a basic exercise program for the mental body. Keep in mind, though, exercising does not replace hygiene. You still need to wash your body. Any exercise program will be more effective if you start with a clean body.

Basic Exercise

When devising an exercise regime it's best to begin with activities that are not too strenuous. For a physical fitness program stretching and conditioning may be recommended. For the mental body we'll start with exercises that stretch and tone your body: Raise the Frequency, Perspective, and Picture-Change.

Raise the Frequency

Sometimes trying to focus the mental body is difficult. It can get stuck in worry, doubt, suspicion, fear, or any number of repetitive thought patterns. Eventually we can't shut it off. This body is prone to becoming unhealthy if it produces low frequency thought-forms, causing it to weaken. As discussed in the previous chapter, whenever a free-floating thought-form encounters another mental body it provokes the same vibration: thought-forms produce thought-forms of the same type, making it easy to get trapped in slow vibration Amplifier Loops. The mental body needs to be toned up so it can resonate with higher frequency thought-forms. In this exercise,[3] attention is focused in the heart to awaken compassion and calm the emotional body, which is usually involved.

Exercise: Raise the Frequency
Application: As needed, to tone the mental body.
Especially helpful for interrupting Amplifier Loops
and to stop stressful thoughts.
Time: 3 minutes

- Find a quiet place in which you can focus without distraction.

- Take a couple of slow, deep breaths.

- Close your eyes and intentionally shift your attention away from an external focus toward an internal focus, awakening your internal senses.

- Allow your physical body to relax.

- Allow your emotional body to relax.

- Allow your mental body to relax.

- Focus your attention in your heart. Visualize a bright yellow flame burning in your heart.

- Clearly visualize the flame. See the flame radiating out. Visualize the halo of light creating a protective circle of light around your body.

- Negative thoughts, like caterpillars, are trying to enter your protective circle of light. When they encounter the light circle they are transformed into beautifully colored moths. Each time a caterpillar comes at you it transforms into a beautiful, colorful winged moth.

- Just as light attracts moths the flame burning brightly in your heart attracts positive thought-forms. Visualize this process for about 1 minute.

- Whenever this feels complete, open your eyes.

Perspective

In conflict situations your mental body is prone to rigidity and contraction. You can get stuck in thinking you are right and the other person is wrong and see only one solution to the problem. Mental body stretching is needed to expand your mental outlook and give perspective. This exercise is helpful in restoring healthy functioning to all seven body types and is useful for clearing up a Signal Scramble, much like pressing the reset button on an electronic device.

Perspective is a mental body exercise that works specifically with a troubling situation. It was designed as a conflict resolution tool[4] and is especially helpful in the aftermath of a disagreement. It can also be used in advance of a stressful situation to prevent conflict from escalating. It engages your conceptual mind and encourages Director's Mode. The exercise consists of five steps in sequential order. Each of the steps represents a particular perspective designed to open the mind:

1) I'm right, you're wrong

2) You're right, I'm wrong

3) Both of us are right and both of us are wrong

4) The issue is not as important as it seems

5) There is truth in all four perspectives

1) I am right and you are wrong. This step is usually very easy. The conviction of rightness is often at the core of any conflict. Allow your mental body to think of all the reasons why you are right and the other person is wrong.

2) You are right and I am wrong. This step requires that you reverse the direction of your thought process completely and assume the position that you are wrong and the other person is right. Stretch your mental body into thinking of all the reasons why this perspective is accurate. Allow plenty of time, as this may be a little difficult at first. You are asked to see the situation from the other person's point of view and to give up your one-sided perspective. Sometimes it may seem impossible to find the merits of the opposing perspective, but stay with it. At the end of the exercise, if you don't like seeing the issue from a different angle, you can go back to your original way of looking at it. You have nothing to lose by doing the exercise. You can gain expanded awareness and, through stretching your mental body, become more open minded. In addition to seeing the strengths of the other person's viewpoint, you also need to find the flaws in your own. This may be equally difficult but every perspective, even your own, has both strengths and weaknesses.

3) Both of us are right and both of us are wrong. This step invites you to view the pros and cons of each perspective and find the commonalities. If you have done a good job in the previous step this one will be relatively easy. Incorporating the two viewpoints helps you see that the issue isn't as black and white as it first seemed. From this step you may find new ways of thinking about the situation, new solutions or fresh ideas. You will also likely discover that the issue is not as big as it once appeared. This leads to the next step.

4) The issue is not as important as it seems. Now that your mental body has stretched out of its limited way of thinking and adopted a broader view, it is easier to see the situation in its proper perspective. Most issues aren't as important as we first think they are. We get so focused on a disagreement that we lose sight of the bigger picture. This leads to the fifth step.

5) There is truth in all four perspectives. The final step in the Perspective exercise reinforces the idea that all four positions have value. There is not just one right and one wrong way of looking at something. Issues are multifaceted and you can stretch your mind to accommodate varied perspectives and create multiple solutions. If nothing else, insight is gained. Your mental body is no longer rigid but has expanded.

To preserve the flow of the exercise, the example below refers to one person, but if your situation involves more than one person Perspective still applies. This is a self-talk exercise.

Exercise: Perspective
Application: As needed, to expand the mental body in times of contraction. Especially useful in disagreements. It helps engage your conceptual mind, encourage Director's Mode, and clear up Signal Scrambles.
Time: 5-10 minutes

- Find a quiet place in which you can focus without distraction.

- Take a couple of slow, deep breaths. Close your eyes and intentionally shift your attention away from an external focus toward an internal focus, awakening your internal senses.

- Allow your physical and emotional bodies to relax.

- Call to mind the conflict situation and complete the following steps in order.

- Step 1: *I am right and you are wrong.* When you have exhausted all possibilities you can move on to the next step.

- Step 2: *You are right and I am wrong.* When you have thought of all the ways in which the other

person is right and you are wrong, you can move on
to the next step.

- Step 3: *Both of us are right and both of us are wrong.*
  Think through this perspective as thoroughly as
  possible, exploring all options, then move to the next
  step.

- Step 4: *The issue is not as important as it seems.*
  Think of all the reasons why this is true. Then move
  on to the last step.

- Step 5: *There is truth in all four perspectives.* Allow
  your mental body to adopt this perspective and lend
  support to it.

- When this feels complete you can open your eyes.

Picture Change

As discussed in the previous chapter, thoughts that you
think about yourself hover around you for quite some time. If you
encounter a distressing situation and think critically about yourself,
the situation can continue to play in your mind and you become
unable to shut it off. This can trigger heavy emotions and create an
Amplifier Loop. In this case, a the following exercise[5] is helpful.

Exercise: Picture Change
Application: As needed, to condition the mental body to
respond in a more positive way. Especially helpful in
times of self-criticism. It enhances Director's Mode
and helps interrupt Amplification Loops.
Time: 3 minutes

- Find a quiet place in which you can focus without distraction.

- Take a couple of slow, deep breaths. Close your eyes and intentionally shift your attention away from an external focus toward an internal focus, awakening your internal senses.

- Allow your physical body to relax.

- Allow your emotional body to relax.

- Allow your mental body to relax.

- Visualize a television in front of you. The screen is displaying a DVD of the stressful situation. Watch the scene, see all of the participants, and see yourself. Pay particular attention to your role in the situation and to your reaction.

- When you have seen enough, remove the DVD and destroy it. You can destroy it in any way you choose.

- Then insert a new DVD. In this version, the situation is playing but you are responding differently, in a better way. Watch the new DVD several times. Find a word or phrase to describe your new response and make a note of it.

- Whenever this feels complete, open your eyes.

This completes the basic program. Once this series of exercises has been mastered you are ready to move on to a more strenuous activity level.

Advanced Training

In the case of the physical body, advanced training often consists of aerobic exercise, core strengthening, and weight lifting. For the mental body we have Breath Focus, Host-Thought, and Receiver exercises to beef up this body's activity level.

Breath Focus

To stay physically fit aerobic exercise such as swimming, jogging, or running improves respiration and enhances the body's use of oxygen. Oxygen for the mental body is found in the space between thoughts. Unlike the physical, the mental body gets more oxygenated with less activity; it gets a chance to breathe in between thoughts. In order to recharge, the mental body needs the quiet spaciousness of an empty mind. This exercise asks you to focus on your breath instead of your thoughts. If thoughts come into your mind, let them pass through. It's as if you are walking down a country road and cars go by but you don't get in a car or interact with them in any way. You just watch them pass by. Observe your thoughts passing by and let them go. Watching your thoughts helps develop your self-observation faculty and enhances Director's Mode.

Exercise: Breath Focus
Application: As needed, to improve overall functioning, and enhance Director's Mode.
Time: 10 minutes
Materials: Clock

- Find a quiet place in which you can focus without distraction.

- Note the start time on your clock. Your session should last about 10 minutes.

- Take a couple of slow, deep breaths. Close your eyes and intentionally shift your attention away from an external focus toward an internal focus, awakening your internal senses.

- Allow your physical body to relax.

- Allow your emotional body to relax.

- Allow your mental body to relax.

- Focus your attention on your breath. Become aware of your breathing so that you can feel yourself breathing from the inside out. Inhale and feel the air as it passes through your nostrils, down your windpipe, into your lungs. Feel it as it passes out again as you exhale.

- Keep your attention focused on your breath.

- If thoughts come into your mind, just observe them passing by, let them go, and return your attention to your breathing.

- When 10 minutes have passed, the exercise is complete. Whenever you are ready open your eyes.

Host-Thought

Core strengthening on the physical level is focused on isolating and working the abdominal muscles that form the inner core of the physical body. On the mental level, the core consists of the conceptual mind. Core strengthening for the mental body involves focusing on and developing your conceptual mind.

The following exercise actively works with the substance of your mental body. It could be regarded as a type of meditation but, to be clear, I am not using the word meditation in any kind of religious sense. It's employed as a general term to describe using your mind in a certain way, namely, to calibrate to higher-frequency inergies. There are many ways to do this. In the case of core strengthening, it is accomplished by focusing your concrete mind on a specific topic and then activating your conceptual mind to receive information about the topic. This involves two abilities. First, it requires quieting your concrete mind enough so that you can get past it in order to access your conceptual mind. Second, it involves the ability to distinguish between concrete and conceptual thoughts.

Many people struggle and eventually stop trying to meditate because they are unable to quiet the concrete mind. Like an overworked secretary, the concrete mind is so accustomed to keeping track of everything that it doesn't know how to stop. If you try to stop it, often it gets threatened and fights to keep its job. This exercise offers a way around that by giving your concrete mind something to do. In this case, it is asked to think about a particular topic, a host-thought. Similar to the intention-host device (IIED) used in the experiments described in Chapter 7, you want to devise and transmit an intention-infused host-thought so it can go forth and attract resonant inergies, like invisible messengers, and bring the information back to you.

You want to direct your concrete mind like a laser to focus on your chosen host-thought; then activate your conceptual mind and remain receptive to the thought-forms you receive. This type of training hones your ability to concentrate. Concentration, remember, is the hallmark of a healthy mental body and a key element in potentizing the effects of your intent.

When choosing a host-thought, pick a topic that you are interested in learning more about. It can be anything you want to understand on a deeper level (i.e., consciousness, color, acceptance, numbers). Similar to intent-setting, it's helpful to think in terms of a quality that you want to awaken in yourself. Have your host-thought ready before you begin the exercise.

Chances are when you first start practicing the exercise, most of the thought-forms you receive will be interference from your concrete mind. For instance, when I first began my host-thought sessions, I chose *love* as my focus. I wanted to truly understand love in a deep way. When I focused my mind on love, hoping for that laser-beam-sharpness-straight-to-the-profound-insights, at first what came in was an influx of Top 40 love songs, followed by love poems from adolescence and, finally, sappy greeting card quotes. This went on for several sessions. Eventually, my concrete mind settled down which allowed some amazing insights to find their way in. You're probably wondering what they were. This brings up an important point: make sure you have a notebook nearby in which to record the results of your session afterwards!

Concentration is the hallmark of a healthy mental body.

It's best to start the exercise by aligning your physical, emotional and mental bodies with the host-thought. This can be accomplished in several ways. If you are visually oriented you might visualize your body cells, emotions, and thoughts giving you an affirmative gesture and then see them lining up with your host-thought. If your orientation is more auditory, you may want to hear them all voicing their agreement. If you are more tactile, you can gently tap your hips (physical), solar plexus (emotions), and head (thoughts), and feel them aligning. Or you can do all three.

Once your bodies are aligned, begin your session by focusing your mind on the chosen host-thought. Pay attention to whatever information you receive, no matter how trivial it may seem. Take a few moments at the end of the exercise to record the results of your session.

Exercise: Host-Thought
Application: As needed, to enhance your conceptual
mind and improve overall functioning.
Time: 10 minutes
Materials: Clock, notebook, chosen host-thought

- Find a quiet place in which you can focus without
  distraction.

- Be in a seated position, as comfortable as possible.

- Note the start time. Your session should last about
  10 minutes.

- Gently close your eyes, take a couple of slow, deep
  breaths and intentionally shift your attention away
  from an external focus toward an internal focus,
  awakening your internal senses.

- Call to mind a topic you wish to focus on (your host-
  thought) with the intent to understand more about it
  and attract resonant thought-forms.

- Align your physical body with your host-thought.

- Align your emotional body with your host-thought.

- Align your mental body with your host-thought.

- Allow your attention to be anchored inside your
  head, in the middle of your head.

- Hold your host-thought at the center of your
  attention and do your best to stay focused exclusively
  on it for the next 10 minutes. If your attention moves
  to something else, gently bring it back to the host-
  thought.

- Be receptive to all thought-forms you receive.

- When 10 minutes have passed, the exercise is finished.

- Take a moment to reflect on your session. Let your physical brain register the thought-forms you have received.

- You can gently become aware of your breathing to help anchor your attention in real time. Feel your feet on the floor. Whenever you are ready open your eyes.

- Use your notebook to record the results of your session.

Receiver

Next we move on to the weight-lifting equivalent of the exercise program. Weight training is done to build muscle mass and improve the strength of the physical body. It can best be accomplished when the body is healthy and conditioned as opposed to when it's weak and out of shape. Similarly, weight training for the mental body is best done when the body has achieved some semblance of toning and strengthening by practicing the previous exercises.

This thought-receiving exercise[6] is designed to help hone your mental body's ability to receive specific thought-forms. Since your brain acts as a receiver, you have a choice about what to attune it to receive. The exercise has two parts, a set-up and the actual exercise. In the set-up you are asked to recruit three friends to help you. They will send you specific thought-forms at predetermined times and you will do your best to receive them.

Exercise: Receiver
Application: As needed, to enhance your mental powers
and improve overall functioning.
Time: 10-15 minutes

The Set-Up

- Ask three of your close friends to participate with
  you in the exercise.

- The exercise will take place at a pre-determined time
  over the course of three days. One of the three friends
  will call you at an appointed time each day.

- The three friends decide beforehand amongst
  themselves who will call you but they do not tell you.
  They may decide that you will get a call from each of
  them, only two of them, or that the same friend will
  call you on each of the three days.

- Together with your friends you decide the exact time
  the "mystery" friend will call you.

- For 10 minutes before the appointed hour, all three
  friends focus their intention on sending you clear,
  concentrated thought-forms of the chosen friend
  who will be calling. Ask them to clearly state the
  friend's name repeatedly, out loud or silently, and to
  form a vivid mental image of the friend and hold it in
  mind. This can also be accomplished by having them
  consistently focus their attention on a photograph of
  the chosen friend and/or a piece of paper with the
  friend's name inscribed on it.

The Exercise

- Your job is to receive the thought-forms.

- Ten minutes before the appointed hour, find a quiet place where you can focus without distraction. Be in a seated position, as comfortable as possible. Take a couple of deep breaths. Gently close your eyes and intentionally shift your attention away from an external focus toward an internal focus, awakening your internal senses.

- Allow your physical body to relax.

- Allow your emotional body to calm.

- Allow your mental body to clear.

- Sharpening your inner senses, do your best to receive the thought-form of the friend who will be calling. Write down any impressions you may receive. Pay attention to subtle details.

- Toward the end of the 10 minutes, "guess" who will be calling. Gather what you have received and write down the name of your chosen friend on a piece of paper.

- When the friend calls, answer the phone and find out if you are right!

The thought-receiving exercise has many variations.[7] You can do an experiment similar to the one above using text messaging or email. Another option is to have a friend stay at home thinking of a grocery shopping list while you go to the store and try to "guess" what's on it.

As you can see, your mental body is quite amazing in its capabilities. It consists of two minds in one, the concrete and the conceptual, that create and magnetize thought-forms. But your inergy constitution doesn't end there. We have one body left to explore, your universal body, that has even greater capacities.

Chapter Nine

Your Universal Body

Every summer researchers, practitioners and educators gather at a professional energy health conference[1] to exchange ideas and techniques. Although the meeting is typically inspirational and useful there was a conference in California one year that I didn't want to attend. I wasn't presenting that year and needed to stay home to finish a writing project. Grappling with various ways to describe a complex concept had put me behind in my writing. Plus, the recent closure of two major airlines that serviced Hawaii sent ticket prices to the mainland skyrocketing. A recent unexpected trip to help out family on the mainland along with some extensive dental work had also taken up precious time and resources. My physical body was tired and I dreaded the thought of flying again. But despite all of this, I just couldn't shake the unwavering sense that I should go to the conference anyway. So I did, promising myself I would diligently write during the six-hour flight back and forth to make up for the lost time.

Shortly after arriving at the conference I began to understand why I was drawn there. I made some very important connections with key people, including a "coincidental" private lunch with the keynote speaker. Also, because I happened to be at the right place at the right time, I was invited to present at the next conference: perfectly synchronized with the release of my new book. Everything was flowing beautifully as if I were riding atop a beneficent wave, being carried by it. But then on the flight back to Maui I sat next to a man who wanted to talk the entire trip. Remembering my promise to write during the flight I tried to avoid conversation. But it was no use. I was in the window seat and he was right next to me for six hours, inquiring about my line of work and asking questions of all kinds. Not wanting to be rude, I kept answering them. In the end, as a direct result of our in-flight conversation, I found an ideal way to describe the complex concept I had been struggling with in my writing, which propelled my project forward in quantum leaps. Yet another confirmation of my choice to make that trip.

So far we've addressed three of the four bodies that comprise your inergy (energy/information) constitution. We discussed the vital body that powers and vitalizes your system. We talked about your emotional body with its inergies of attraction and repulsion that govern your feelings and desires. We covered your mental body, how thought-forms behave, and the power of your intent. However, what happens when you don't feel like doing something—physically or emotionally—and you actually intend *not* to do it; but you get the sense you should do it anyway, and it turns out to be exactly what you needed, as in the story above? Where does that intuitive "sense to do it" come from? Why do some people seem to have it and others don't? How could "that sense" know in advance what you should do? What invisible forces could arrange for the synchronistic timing and movement of events that would cause particular people to be in exact positions at precise moments to bring about outcomes such as those described above?

Enter the universal body. This body occupies the highest frequency range of the inergy continuum—the universal level. Four important qualities characterize this body and distinguish it from any of your other bodies:

- It contains ultra-high frequency inergies that can be difficult to discern.

- Its inergies are extremely high-powered, capable of significant effects on the lower frequency (more dense) levels.

- Its inergies are essentially unitive in nature.

- Its inergies are mobile and limitless allowing them to travel anywhere without known bounds.

Within the realm of ordinary physics high frequency energies exist outside of our normal perception but we are well aware of their effects. A simple example is a dog whistle. Most people can't hear the high-pitched sound but when a dog responds to the whistle we can see its effects. Along the same lines, high frequency vibrations are known to reorganize physical matter. A microwave oven produces waves that vibrate at a rate of about 2.4 billion times per second, a very high frequency. That invisible force causes material substance to change form: the food goes from raw to cooked. Sounding a particularly high note can set up a vibration that shatters a glass. In like manner, because they are vibrating at ultra-high frequencies, the invisible inergies of the universal body are potent, capable of causing significant changes in lower frequency levels.

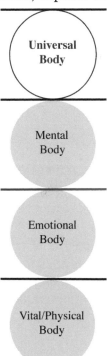

In terms of the universal, just as with the vital body, less is more: the less densified the inergy, the more potency it has. This can be a difficult concept to grasp, especially since it goes against much of what we know about physical reality. Massive, hard objects appear to be stronger and to have more impact. If you want to break a glass you use a large hammer, not your singing voice. However, in the world of inergies, the higher the frequency, the subtler the vibration, the more potency it has. The ultra-high frequency inergies of the universal level bring us closer to the level of cause, whereas material substance is at the level of effect.

Your universal body occupies the universal level of experience and is positioned next to your mental body. Thus, most inergies from the universal body are made available to you via your mental body. The universal body works behind-the-scenes in powerful yet imperceptible ways. Because of the subtly of this body, its inergies can be difficult to detect. Discerning them requires you to be receptive to extremely elusive influences. It's necessary to quiet down your physical, emotional, and mental bodies to facilitate the process. Otherwise the rarefied inergies of the universal body can be easily missed or overshadowed by the denser, more obvious bodies.

Limitations of Language

Not only are the inergies of the universal body difficult to discern, they are also challenging to describe in words due to the limitations of the English language. Historically, Western cultures have supported an artificial split between the seen and unseen worlds. The visible world belonged to science and the invisible was the domain of religion. As a result there are not adequate commonly used words to describe the subtleties and complexities of the unseen realms. We end up borrowing words from other languages but that poses its own problems since many of those words don't translate well or they tend to have connotations that can be alienating or hard to grasp.

Keeping in mind these limitations, it may be easier to understand your universal body according to what it is not. It is not your other bodies. You have a vital body that powers your physical body and brings it to life; you have emotional and mental bodies as well. But you are not your vitality, movement, emotions, or thoughts. You have feelings, actions, and ideas but this is not you. If we peel away the layers of your bodies we get closer to the essence of who you really are. You are not your physical body, you are the one who directs and moves your body. You initiate the activity. You are not your emotions, you are the one who experiences emotions. You are not your thoughts, you are the one who thinks the thoughts. The list could go on. You are not your possessions. You are not your work. You are not your past, or your experiences. You are much more than that. You are not your loved ones. You are not anyone else. You are not the roles you play in society. You are not anything that exists outside of you. You are not a thing. You are *no-thing*. What, then, are you?

Consciousness

As we continue up the inergy continuum from physical matter to higher frequency levels we encounter the universal body and come closer to the essence of what you really are. In contrast to your other bodies, which are confined to their particular frequency domains, your universal body is mobile and limitless. It can extend into your physical body but your physical body cannot extend to the universal; it is limited to the material realm. The same is true for your other bodies. You can have feelings and thoughts about the universal but you cannot actually experience it with those bodies. They are limited to their respective domains whereas your universal body is not. It has no boundaries. It accomplishes this through consciousness. Just as the substance of the physical body is matter, the emotional body is feelings, and the mental body is thoughts, the substance of the universal body is consciousness. When your universal body is healthy, your consciousness is expansive and continuous. When it's unhealthy, your consciousness is contracted or fragmented.

In this context we are not talking about waking versus sleeping. Consciousness is an ultra-high frequency inergy that originates from the universal level and brings unity to whatever it encounters. As such, it is inherently transformative and healing, repairing fragmentation and restoring wholeness. It ranges from expansive unity consciousness at the universal level to highly focused attention at the personal level. Thus, when you bring conscious awareness to your inergy bodies (vital/physical, emotional, mental, and universal) you are transforming and healing them, uniting them and making them whole. The exercises throughout this book have been designed to help with this. Now we are addressing the universal body from which consciousness itself originates. This requires that consciousness become aware of itself, much of what this chapter is about.

Like your inergy constitution, consciousness is a continuum. It originates from the universal level and extends to your other bodies. It has five gradations, from lowest to highest frequency:

- Selective
- Individual
- Collective
- Intuitive
- Unity

Unity consciousness is the highest frequency of our inergy constitution. It allows for the experience of essential oneness. It is the mother lode, the superset. From there, consciousness refracts into collective consciousness, which is the aggregate of all individual consciousnesses. From the collective level, consciousness then individuates into intuition. Intuitive consciousness allows for profound insights and the ability to see behind things. Consciousness further refracts into your individual consciousness, amassed over the span of your lifetime. From your personal consciousness it individuates via what you pay attention to in each and every moment. Yes, your personal attention span is an offshoot of unity consciousness. Although each of these dimensions is discreet, there is reciprocity among them; they mutually influence each other. Let's explore them in more detail, starting with the most individuated.

Selective Consciousness

Selective consciousness refers to your individual awareness. It is determined by where you choose to place your attention. Selection is intrinsic to the process of perception. In order to interface with the world you have to select what to pay attention to because it's not possible to take in everything. There's just too much and attention is simply too limited. In any given moment you are swimming in a sea of stimuli. You attend to certain aspects while ignoring others. Awareness is confined to a particular focus depending on what you choose to pay attention to.

At the start of this book, in Chapter 2, we discussed your internal senses, attention being one of them. We talked about how inergy is responsive to attention; that what you focus your attention on is changed at a fundamental level. Called the *observer effect* in quantum physics, the mere act of observation, of bringing your attention to something, changes it. This happens because your personal awareness is a derivative of unity consciousness, an ultra-high frequency inergy that has potent effects. Selection involves free will. You have the ability to freely choose

Your personal attention span is an offshoot of unity consciousness.

what to attend to and what to omit. That choice is always yours to make; no one can take that away from you. However, there are many factors that influence your selection process: family, peer, media, cultural, religious, political, and commercial influences, to name just a few. Although some of these factors are extremely powerful and insidious, you still always have a choice. Never forget this.

When your universal body is healthy you are consciously and freely choosing what to pay attention to on an ongoing basis. In each moment you are aware of where you focus. When your universal body is unhealthy, the selection process is unconscious, automatic, and/or largely determined by outside influences. Selection is such an intrinsic part of our ability to perceive reality that we often don't notice it at all. We don't realize that in each moment we are choosing what to attend to, what potential we will actualize. It's important to take an active role in the selection process because where you choose to focus your attention, as we will soon see, has profound implications for yourself and for others.

Individual Consciousness

Individual consciousness refers to your personal consciousness. It is the aggregate of your individual thoughts, feelings, and sensitivities. It brings continuity to your experiences. It's the glue that holds your life, in all of its complexities, together bringing meaning to a vast array of events. Without consciousness your experiences would be completely random. You would have to repeat and relearn everything every time you awoke because it's not memory that allows you to grow and learn. Memory merely brings recognition. Computers and calculators have memory. They can be programmed to recognize and store information, but they lack consciousness. Consciousness gives meaning. It allows you to connect the dots of your personal experiences in a unique and meaningful way.

Consciousness extends out into the world via individuated awareness-laced experiences; this awareness is then deposited into the larger repository of consciousness. In essence, your individual consciousness is the sum-total of your awareness. It's like a pool of water that is fed through the individual tributaries of your awareness. As a dimension of the universal body, consciousness itself is vibrating at ultra-high frequency and therefore has cause-effect capabilities.

The Causal Effect

Consciousness causes changes. Your other bodies are affected by the inergy of consciousness and reconfigure accordingly. This phenomenon is most vivid in people with multiple personalities where the same individual can have widely differing physical attributes depending upon which personality is activated.[2] One personality can have brown eyes, perfect vision, and be diabetic while another personality of the same individual can have green eyes, no diabetes, and be nearsighted. Even allergies and EEG brainwaves can differ. Indeed, the new field of epigenetics reveals that your individual consciousness actively controls not only your body cells but also your genes.[3] As renowned author and physician

Deepak Chopra has said: "different consciousnesses have different metabolisms."

Below is a sampling of various levels of consciousness as calibrated by notable author and psychiatrist David Hawkins.[4] Notice that higher frequency states are more inclusive, aligned with unity consciousness, while lower states are more separative.

High Frequency States

Level	Calibration
Peace	600
Love	500
Reason	400
Acceptance	350
Willingness	310
Neutrality	250

Low Frequency States

Level	Calibration
Pride	175
Desire	125
Fear	100
Grief	75
Apathy	50
Guilt	30

From the perspective of your universal body, it's not so important *what* you do. *Why* you do it matters most. What is your interior motivation? What state of consciousness are you bringing to that experience? Is it aligned with unity or separateness? Your consciousness determines the experience and has the strongest effects. Let's say you are cooking dinner for a couple of friends. Your state of consciousness in doing this will determine (i.e., *create*) the experience. Are you cooking out of love for them (high frequency, unitive inergy)? Are you motivated by pride because you just learned a great new recipe that you want to show-off (moderately low, relatively separative inergy)? Or are you cooking out of guilt because they invited you over last month and now you feel obligated to return the favor although you don't want to (even lower frequency inergy)? Each of these states will produce a qualitatively different experience that is predetermined by you. You determine the experience—you *cause* the experience—by the state of your individual consciousness.

The Two-Way Effect

But it doesn't stop there. Consciousness is two-way. You contribute to your individual consciousness through your awareness; but you then draw from it as your individual consciousness, in turn, conditions your awareness. It becomes the filter through which you view things, the lens coloring your experiences and shaping what you pay attention to and what gets missed. It's impossible to truly apprehend the totality of any experience because reality is too vast and individual awareness is limited. Thus, we get only snippets of reality. What you perceive versus what gets omitted is determined by the condition of your universal body, or more specifically, the condition of your individual consciousness.

A Colombian friend who lives in the capital city of Bogota once spent a summer deep in the Amazon rainforest with the indigenous people. They would hunt for a particular insect, rather large in size, that provided a major food source. The insects lived on the leaves of certain trees that were abundant in the rainforest. My friend tried to join them in a hunt but was not very helpful, as he literally could not see the insects even when they were in plain view. All he could see were layers upon layers of green leaves in varying hues. There was nothing wrong with his physical eyes; his inability to perceive the insects was reflective of his individual consciousness. Because he spent his whole life in the city his consciousness was influenced by those experiences. That was the "pool" he had to draw from and, as such, he was unable to see the forest food. In this respect we can again see how consciousness creates reality. The insects literally did not exist for him. We shape our individual consciousness and our consciousness shapes us, meaning, how you see is what you get.

The Elastic Effect

When the Amazonians repeatedly and painstakingly pointed out the creatures, eventually my friend was able to make them out more easily. His individual consciousness expanded to the extent that he could readily perceive the food-source that was previously invisible to him and, in turn, his reality transformed. His world became bigger. This signifies a healthy universal body.

It's also possible for individual consciousness to contract. When this happens, reality shrinks. Take Jenna, for example. She fell in love with Ken and soon her whole world revolved around him. She moved in with him and now takes care of his house, his children from a previous marriage, his custody battle, his meals, his clothes, his health, and his issues at work. Her consciousness is contracted. Derek is another example. He is fixated on information. He is either interacting with his computer, his cell phone, or a book. If he is without access to an information source, he craves it and begins to feel uncomfortable. To quote Deepak Chopra again, "consciousness shrinks to fit." If you hyper-focus your awareness on something or someone, your individual consciousness will contract accordingly. Since reality is defined by what you focus on, reality contracts as well. This is the sign of an unhealthy universal body. If a hyper-focused state is sustained over time, it becomes toxic to the inergy bodies. The next chapter contains exercises to help detoxify.

Your individual consciousness is not meant to be fixed. It is elastic, an ever-changing dynamic process. When consciousness contracts, reality becomes limited and fragmented. When it expands, your reality becomes richer and fuller, potentially infinite.

Collective Consciousness

But it's not really consciousness that expands or contracts; it's our ability to access it. Consciousness itself is not limited;

individual consciousness is. We tend to think of consciousness as being confined to the brain. It is not. Consciousness is collective. It is more than an aggregate of *your* past and present awareness that reciprocally conditions your future awareness. Consciousness is a dynamic field of *all* awareness. Everyone contributes to and draws from the composite collectivity of consciousness; it is not confined to any particular individual or any one place.

There is a growing body of research that substantiates this. Take, for example, the pupillary response, the involuntary response of your eye pupils to dilate or contract when exposed to positive or negative stimuli. Recent research on consciousness shows that your pupils will respond in the exact same manner when the positive and negative stimuli are *hidden* from the eye.[5] Although the images are not visible your pupils still respond accordingly,

How you see
is what you get.

as though the images were in plain sight. Clearly your system is tapping into something beyond the physical realm, beyond your ordinary senses. Similar findings are evident with the human heart, which has been shown to consistently and appropriately respond to random generated positive or negative images even *before* you are exposed to them.[6] The collective consciousness is an ultra-high frequency energy/information structure that we are tuned in to. It exists as a universal inergy field that we simultaneously contribute to and are conditioned by.

The World Wide Web, and the Internet that supports it, are helpful in illustrating how this works. Like consciousness, the Net itself does not exist in material form. It consists of bits and bytes (binary digits) of information. It requires hardware and software to function just as consciousness requires a physical body (hardware) along with mental and emotional bodies (software) in order to function.

Like consciousness, the Internet is not confined to one location. It is pervasive. Sitting in front of my computer one typical day while paying bills, ordering gifts, exchanging emails/instant messages, surfing the Web, and registering to vote, it occurred to me how dependent on the Internet I had become. I wondered how I could function, not to mention the rest of the industrialized world, if the Net went down for any length of time. So I asked a computer engineer about the probability of this happening. He said it would be impossible because the Internet does not exist in any specific location. Rather, it consists of countless servers positioned throughout the planet. If a server goes down in one location there are enough others still functioning to sustain the Net. In similar fashion, everyone is constantly contributing to consciousness. It does not exist in any one location but is omnipresent. It is dynamic, pervasive, and ever-expanding. There is virtually no end to it. Like an enormous Internet, the consciousness web is potentially limitless.

The Internet is comprised of individual information streams from all over the world. People are continually accessing it, contributing to it, drawing from it. It represents a singular, yet collective effort. Individuals shape the content of the Net through their personal contributions to it and, in turn, are shaped by it. Just like the Internet anyone, anywhere, at any time can (and does) contribute to the collective consciousness. In a two-way effect, you shape it through your individual contributions to it and you are simultaneously conditioned by it.

Intuitive Consciousness

The vast storehouse of information from the collective consciousness is available to you through intuitive consciousness. Just as everyone has eyes to see, we are all intuitive. Intuition is not something you are born with or without, nor is it a special gift. It is available to us all. In fact, it is a relatively common capacity[7] that can be enhanced with a little focused awareness and practice. The only difference between an intuitive and non-intuitive person is the two have used their selective consciousness differently. In other words, they have paid attention to different frequencies. There are various kinds of intuition so it's important to make a distinction between two basic types: gut-level and higher-level intuition. Higher-level intuition is associated with the universal body whereas gut-level intuition is not.

Gut-Level Intuition

Gut-level intuition refers to inergy coming in from the emotional frequency band. Because of the close proximity of the emotional to the physical body, gut-level intuition, as the name implies, is experienced in the gut. When the inergies come in, sensations will often be felt in the solar plexus area. They could be experienced as heaviness, queasiness, or butterflies. Let's say you have a date with a new acquaintance, Chris, in a few days. After a recent phone conversation to finalize plans you realize you have an uneasy feeling in your gut. On the phone you learned that Chris travels a lot for work and this is exactly what caused the demise of your previous relationship. Your ex fell in love with a travel partner on a business trip. A feeling of dread lingers in your abdominal area. Gut-level intuition contains energy and information from your emotional body. It will tell you what you are afraid of, hurt by, or excited about.

Gut-level intuition provides valuable guidance in life so it's important not to shut down this channel of information. However, if you act only according to your gut you may be in for quite a roller coaster ride. Gut-level intuition will register excitement and anxiety, attraction and repulsion, often about the very same thing. You can move toward the excitement but avoid the anxiety and end up going nowhere. In the example above, after the initial excitement about Chris, your gut would tell you to be very cautious. You may be inclined to cancel the date for fear that Chris's traveling would cause problems in a relationship. Although the traveling is an important consideration, at some point it's necessary to acknowledge the fear and move forward anyway instead of allowing the fear to determine your actions. Chris is not your ex. If you frequently avoid situations out of fear, you can rob yourself of potentially rewarding opportunities and valuable life experience. In an effort to stay emotionally safe, your world remains small. Chris could end up being the love of your life but gut-level intuition would not tell you that. This is where higher-level intuition is more helpful.

Higher-Level Intuition

Higher-level intuition refers to inergy coming from the universal level. In contrast to gut-level, higher-level intuition does not register in the gut and is not emotionally-based. Because of the close proximity of the mental to the universal body, higher-level intuition comes in through the mental body as a pure, clear knowing. You don't know how you know it or why you know it, you have not been thinking about it or trying to figure it out. You just know it. This kind of inergy usually gives guidance of a higher order, as universal inergies originate from a higher frequency range.

Although higher-level intuition is not emotionally-based it can sometimes evoke strong feelings. Let's look at an example. While happily residing in the San Francisco Bay area, seemingly out of nowhere came the intuitive insight that I move to Maui. I had not been thinking about moving. In fact, residing in the Bay area was the fulfillment of a life-long dream so I was quite happy with my home. But three years after moving there the faintest of thoughts floated in and whispered *Maui*. Then, synchronistically, a friend invited me to visit the island. Of course, I accepted and, like so many others, fell in love with Hawaii. While enjoying my holiday in paradise another synchronistic invitation came—free housing on Maui in exchange for a few hours of work each month. How could I refuse? But when I chose to accept, it touched off fear in my emotional body. Following the higher-level intuition meant leaving a nice job and good friends in California to live in a place where I didn't know anyone and had no income source. My emotional body and gut certainly had a reaction to that! But I chose to move anyway and the results were overwhelmingly positive.

Many of us are in touch with gut-level intuition but not so aware of the subtleties of the higher-level. Often when the higher frequency inergies do come in, because they're so subtle, we tend to miss or ignore them. The challenge is to quiet down the other bodies enough to discern the higher frequency inergy and then have the courage to follow it. The previous chapters and exercises in this book were designed to help with this. By creating healthy inergy bodies you can be more receptive to higher-level intuition, along with other universal inergies, and reconfigure your life in significant ways. When your universal body is healthy, you have easy access to higher-level intuition. When it is unhealthy, you do not.

Intuitive consciousness affords powerful guidance in life. It may take the form of a subtle but pervasive sensibility about something. It may also take the form of sudden insights, epiphanies, and "a-ha" experiences in which something that previously evaded your awareness suddenly becomes clear and accessible. Intuitive consciousness gives you a broader perspective, the ability to see the bigger picture, to see behind things. It opens a window into the collective consciousness. But it doesn't stop there.

Unity Consciousness

We not only have access to the collective consciousness via intuition, we also contribute to consciousness. This two-way process has universal effects. What you contribute to the collectivity determines not only your future experiences but those of others as well. We are all connected. The Hundredth Monkey Effect is a profound example of this.[8] The Japanese monkey, Macaca fuscata, was studied over a period spanning more than 30 years. In 1952, on the island of Koshima, the monkeys were being fed sweet potatoes that scientists dropped in the sand. But the monkeys didn't like their potatoes with sand, so they would painstakingly pick it off. Then one day a young female named Imo discovered she could wash the potatoes in a nearby stream. She taught this shortcut to her mother and her playmates. In typical monkey-see-monkey-do fashion the learned behavior spread and by 1958 many monkeys in the colony had adopted the technique.

Then something incredible happened, as the story goes. When critical mass had been reached, when the proverbial "hundredth monkey" had learned the behavior, monkeys in at least five different colonies on neighboring islands spontaneously began washing their potatoes without ever having been shown how to do it. By virtue of being monkeys, the neighboring primates were tapped into the frequency of "collective monkey consciousness" and the new information immediately became available to them through no effort on their part. Similar events have been documented in other species as well as in humans.[9]

Profound evidence of this unity is found in "technologies of consciousness," practices in which trained meditators tune-in to the unified field of consciousness and work with it in intentional ways. These techniques have been successfully implemented to reduce war, terrorism, and social conflict.[10] They have been shown to turn-off violence in the Middle East[11] and reduce crime in 47 cities, including a 25% drop in violent crime in Washington DC.[12] Consciousness is a unified field constantly uploading, reconfiguring, and downloading information that affects us all; we are all connected.

Unity is Real

Unity is not just a flowery feel-good idea; it is a fact. Atoms—the very essence of life—are not made of material substance as was previously thought. Therefore neither are we. Despite outward appearances of separateness, we are all one, interconnected via a vast inergy matrix. In 1964 Irish physicist John Stewart Bell devised a mathematical theorem that is often referred to as the most profound in all of science.[13] Bell proved reality is nonlocal, or nonseparable. His theorem is remarkable because it is not a theory or speculation, it is a mathematical proof that explains reality itself, not appearances or perceptions of reality. Bell's proof has been experimentally verified and shows there is a profound holistic interconnectedness that permeates all of existence. The dominant concept of reality as separate objects and individuals is just not accurate.

Unity is the true nature of reality. We simply are not conscious of it; therefore it is not actualized. It exists as potential. The actualization of unity happens through the expansion of consciousness, as *the very substance of life does not fully come to life until it interacts with consciousness.* At the subatomic level, matter only exists as potentials or tendencies until it encounters consciousness. Reality is literally co-created by us through what we observe, what we pay attention to. When we infuse something with consciousness, it transforms. When a child is born its consciousness is very limited. An infant can be fascinated or even frightened by the movement of its own hand, not realizing the hand is theirs. Then one day, consciousness expands. The child becomes aware of its hand and the extension of consciousness into the hand means the appendage is no longer seen as separate. Unity is restored. Consciousness grows, eventually pervading the entire physical body allowing the child to move about as a unified whole. The expansion of consciousness continues and more coherence is attained. Unity is actualized through the recognition of essential wholeness.

Unity consciousness gives you the lived experience of oneness, or what has been described as beingness itself. At the level of unity you do not merely *observe* a flower in its pure form, you *become one* with the flower. You do not so much *see* a blade of grass, you *are* the blade of grass, along with everything and everyone else. You do not see the other person you *are* that person. That tree. The planet. The galaxy. The universe. Unity prevails. It becomes evident that consciousness and love are essentially one and the same.

Nothing is Good or Bad

It's pleasant to ponder on this kind of unity when it comes to flowers and trees and things you like. It is equally important to realize that when you reach this level of unity consciousness you also experience that you *are* the annoying neighbor, the critical boss, the terrorist, and the serial killer. It is not about *becoming one* with things, it's that you *already are* one with everything. There is no separation. Only unity.

We are taught to think of the world as separated into good and bad, a kind of yin-yang that maintains balance. We are told we wouldn't know the good without the bad. With this kind of dual thinking, in order to be good, the bad has to exist outside of us. We are good; the serial killer is bad. However, *nothing is good or bad*, we make it so. Reality exists as potential that is actualized by our consciousness. The two cannot be separated. If there is evil in the world, there is evil in consciousness, yours and mine, because we are all one. Evil does not exist out in the world separate from us. There is no such thing as separation. Each of us is a combination of good and evil. But dual thinking, such as good and evil, is itself separative.

To echo the words of former Czech President Vaclav Havel, the problems in the world were not created out in the world, they are problems of the mind. Let's say you wake up tomorrow morning and somehow everything is transformed—no more war, pollution, poverty, racism, oppression, sexism, or persecution—no more problems of any kind. In a very short time they would all come back because the problems are not out there in the world; they are inside each of us. They are problems of consciousness. If it shows up out in the world, it already exists inside of us, in our consciousness.

If you had diabetes and your arm got an infection you would not condemn the arm as evil, cut it off and destroy it. You would treat the diabetes, care for the infection, and do everything to save the arm. The serial killer is like your arm. He is an essential part of you. And me. We are one. He is an indicator of the condition of our collective consciousness; as such, only through a change in consciousness can the true problem be solved. Good, in this light, is anything that takes us in the direction of unity, of essential wholeness and profound interconnection.

The Problem of Separation

We all have a universal body and are therefore capable of accessing unity consciousness as a way of life. So why not do this? Why don't we abide in the awareness of our interconnectedness at all times? Why do we feel so isolated and alone sometimes? Why do we act in ways that are harmful to each other when in reality we are all one? To answer this question, let's travel to the middle of the

Pacific ocean . . . deep, expansive . . . teeming with life . . . unified, all-encompassing. Here we meet a wave. We'll call him Kai.

Kai emerged from the ocean one day, popped his head above the waterline, and was curious about what he saw. From his new vantage point as an individual wave he could see many things that were previously invisible. He could see the vast horizon, he could see the sky above, the water below, and he could see other waves. Kai was a bit overwhelmed by all of this and at times he felt vulnerable. So he would stay very still and hope to go unnoticed. When he got tired of that he'd move around a bit. Eventually it felt safe to be so exposed. He grew to like moving as a wave. He loved the sense of freedom and independence.

Kai learned that if he moved faster he could gain momentum and grow bigger quite effortlessly. Now he could see even more—birds flying, dolphins jumping, and whales breaching. He eventually joined with another wave. Together they produced small waves. They grew and Kai grew. He became older and bigger and traveled faster. Soon Kai was towering over the ocean. He loved this feeling. He could move with the cruise ships, sailing yachts, and ocean liners. He became bigger, stronger and more powerful. He gained even more momentum and gathered even more experiences. He began moving with a fast crowd, looking for new adventures, when suddenly something strange rose up abruptly on the horizon. He didn't know what it was but he was advancing toward it with such momentum that he couldn't avoid a head-on collision. It appeared to be a massive solid object. Kai panicked. At the last moment he caught a clear glimpse of it. It was what everyone had warned him about—the shoreline. Oh dear god, he was about to lose everything! Terrified, he tried to avoid it but there was nothing he could do. He let out a blood curdling sound and slammed into the shore. And transformed back into the ocean water that was his essence . . .

Like Kai, we are all individual waves moving in an ocean of inergy. And, like Kai, we get caught-up in our individuated forms and forget what we really are. We believe we are separate but we are not. Separateness is indicative of an unhealthy universal body.

Sometimes we catch glimpses of the essential oneness. This happens frequently when the universal body is healthy, less frequently or not at all if this body is unhealthy.

The universal body compels us to bring unity consciousness to all aspects of life, to use our will to unify because we comprehend the interconnectedness of all and act from that state of consciousness. The universal body, consciousness, is the great synthesizing force that derives unity out of fragmentation and propels us forward in this direction. Our individual thoughts, feelings, actions and awareness directly impact others via the universal body. We are, therefore, called upon to make choices accordingly: to make every action a conscious action; every feeling a conscious feeling; every thought a conscious thought. To use free will to choose unity, and be responsible for our participation in the essential oneness. Proper care of your universal body, as outlined in the next chapter, can help make the way a little easier.

Chapter Ten

Steps to a Healthy Universal Body

The universal body is so subtle and discreet that it is easily over-looked. It's not prone to weight problems like the emotional body. Nor is it customarily overworked like the mental body. With Western cultures, in particular, the physical, emotional and mental bodies take precedence leaving the universal body relatively underdeveloped. For the most part the universal body is simply passed by. When it is acknowledged, this enigmatic body is often misunderstood and therefore not properly cared for.

Discerning the needs of the universal body can be challenging due to the many paradoxes inherent in its nature. The universal body is elusive because its inergy is difficult to discern without quieting down the other bodies, yet it is always present in those bodies via consciousness. This body exists as potential that is relatively unactualized, yet this latent potential pervades everything in existence. The universal body manifests itself through your individual physical body, yet it connects everyone and everything in the metaphysical web of life. The universal body is extremely subtle because of its ultra-high frequency range, yet that very attribute imbues it with potent causal inergies that have far reaching effects. With so many inherent paradoxes it's no wonder this body's needs are hard to understand.

When your universal body is healthy, your individual consciousness is ever-expanding. When it's unhealthy consciousness is in a latent form, much like a newborn infant, imbued with enormous potential that can only be fully actualized through fostering care. Thus, the universal body doesn't require a special diet like the emotional body, nor does it need an exercise regimen like the mental body. The universal body requires proper upbringing that nurtures its development, creating the right conditions for the expansion of consciousness.

The full development of your universal body is dependent on the health of your other inergy bodies. The three bodies—vital/physical, emotional, and mental combined—comprise your ego. Because the universal body pervades the ego via consciousness, it can only fully develop when the ego bodies are consciously attended to and well maintained. If your vital, emotional or mental bodies are unhealthy, the universal body's growth is impeded because it cannot express itself through these unhealthy vehicles. So, an important way to support your universal body is to consciously maintain the health of your ego bodies. The exercises in the previous chapters were designed to help with this.

When the universal body is developed it acts as the primary control center. Its signals transmit clearly and resist distortion. Like a searchlight beaming through a storm, unimpeded by the wind and rain, a healthy universal body radiates consciousness indiscriminately and illuminates everything while remaining unhindered by anything in its path. It clearly guides the way. Your ego bodies, when healthy, align with the universal and there is at-one-ment. You are able to see deep, high and wide, to consistently hold the bigger picture, to clearly apprehend the many dimensions of reality. You are able to truly and fully live your life's purpose, which inherently involves attending to the interconnectedness of all. Every moment is an opportunity for unity.

The key is to maintain balanced growth between your universal body and ego bodies. A newly developing universal body is easily overshadowed by the needs of the ego bodies. Because of this, we can become overly protective of this body and want to isolate from the outside world to foster its growth. We may mistakenly think the universal body can only flourish in a controlled environment, with outside stimulation kept to a minimum, say, in a monastery or cloister. In fact, the universal body does not reach its full potential divorced from the real world where the activities of the other inergy bodies are engaged. It cannot mature and achieve unity consciousness in isolation, disconnected from life. The universal body pervades your ego bodies via consciousness; therefore it can only fully develop when the vital, emotional and mental bodies are consciously developed. This necessitates living in the world with others. A mature universal body is nonseparative, limitless. It is concerned with expanding consciousness, bringing unity consciousness to all aspects of life, for to disconnect from any aspect of life is to separate from all.

Full development of the universal body is dependent upon the ego bodies. Consciousness needs a strong container in order to be effective in the world. Your ego bodies form this container. Thus, your ego bodies need to be strong and healthy, not neglected or discounted. But balanced growth is essential. If the growth of the ego bodies relative to the universal is disproportionate, two conditions emerge. If your ego bodies are strong and your universal body is undeveloped, the inergies of the universal body can easily be distorted and misused by your ego. This results in a Duping Syndrome,[1] explained below. The strong ego bodies want their way so they take over and can misuse ultra-high frequency universal inergies for their own purposes. Conversely, if your ego bodies are weak and your universal body is strong, the weak ego bodies can get easily hypnotized by the potent inergies of your universal body resulting in a Trancing Syndrome.[2] Let's look at the Duping Syndrome first.

The Duping Syndrome

Duping happens when the universal body is in its infancy, so to speak. In the early stages of development this body's inergy range is limited, giving it a smaller sphere of influence in your inergy constitution. When your ego bodies are strong and healthy and operating without the universal body's conditioning inergies, they are left to their own devices. There is little to temper and guide them toward wholeness. Ego inergies easily pass off as universal inergies because the ego bodies cannot tell the difference. In a case of mistaken identity, the ego bodies get duped. Low frequency "feel-good" inergies become substituted for unity consciousness.

When duping happens, instead of consciousness expanding, the lower bodies seek out bliss-type experiences that they believe to be experiences of the universal body. They are drawn to altered states of consciousness, drug-induced highs, or emotional intensity, and mistake these ego-gratifying experiences for unity consciousness. Duping can take many forms. It's impossible to list them all because, ultimately, only you can determine whether you are duping or not. Remember, from the perspective of the universal

To separate from any aspect of life is to separate from all.

body, it doesn't matter *what* you do; it matters *why* you do it. Only you know what is truly motivating you, what state of consciousness you are bringing to an experience. Are you driven by the needs of the ego bodies or by the universal will-to-unity? Anything that you are habitually engaged in, feels good to the ego bodies, and does not serve unity consciousness could qualify as duping. This doesn't mean the expansion of consciousness has to feel bad; it simply means that feeling good or comfortable for the sake of the ego bodies is not the determining factor. Again, it's not so important what you do, why you do it matters most.

Some indicators that the Duping Syndrome may be at play include over-focusing on the material plane, hunger for power, relaxation addiction, or misuse of inergy for personal gains. Duping is a trap that can seriously derail development of the universal body. The underdeveloped body gets ensnared in the desires of strong ego bodies and its identity gets confused. When it's more mature, the universal body is not particularly interested in whether something is appealing to the ego bodies. It does not desire to discount or neglect the ego bodies; it is simply not concerned with indulging them. Instead of focusing on gratifying the ego bodies, the universal body is involved with actualizing unity consciousness on all levels. A mature universal body directs the ego bodies to align with this. It's concerned with taking responsibility and doing its part in the profound wholeness. Next let's look at the Trancing Syndrome, which has different origins but can be equally debilitating to the growth of the universal body.

The Trancing Syndrome

When trancing happens the universal body is overdeveloped relative to the ego bodies. In this case, the inergies of the universal body are relatively strong and far ranging but they get distorted by underdeveloped ego bodies. The universal frequency band is ultra-high, and therefore potent, causing the needs of the universal body to be advanced at the expense of the lower frequency bodies. The inergy of unity consciousness—and other attributes associated with the universal body—are highly alluring to the frail ego bodies. Because they are in a weakened state, they capitulate.

Instead of bringing forth their inergies in support of the universal body, the ego bodies become passive and have little to offer. An unhealthy emotional body is readily seduced by the warm-fuzzy feelings associated with unity consciousness and universal love. Similarly, a weak mental body is susceptible to the idea of interconnectedness. It easily latches on to such a notion and elevates it to a lofty ideal. When distortions like these happen, the ego bodies become hypnotized into a kind of trance. They go unconscious and repeat the same idealistic mantra (i.e., *I just need to love more, I just need to love more*). Their expressions are not fully manifest and their needs are not truly addressed. Instead, they are subordinated for the sake of the ideal. The trancing of the lower bodies creates a domino effect. It can perpetuate unhealthy ego bodies, lead to a stunted universal body, and contribute to a devitalized state that could eventually render you ineffectual.

Let's say Chelsea believes in unconditional love. She knows this is a universal truth. That's why, when her boss mistreats her, her boyfriend neglects her, and her friends take advantage of her, she habitually turns the other cheek. She is compulsively nice. She doesn't really register physical stress, emotional exhaustion, or mental confusion. Her physical, emotional, and mental bodies are mesmerized by the ideal of unconditional love and are compelled to keep reminding her of that. Indeed, she has been reminding herself for so long that her ego bodies are programmed accordingly. But her life does not reflect unconditional love. Instead, she feels increasingly burdened and tested at every turn. She is chronically tired and struggles with physical ailments.

In another instance, Jason believes in justice as a universal ideal. He is committed to helping the disadvantaged through a project in his community. In addition to his day job he works evenings and weekends pouring over legal documents for the cause. He was making payments on his five-year-old car when a key player in the project told him she needed a car. In an act of divine inspiration Jason gave his car to her in support of the cause. Then he had to buy a new car. A healthy emotional body would have registered anxiety over amassing more debt and a healthy mental body would have calculated that he simply could not afford double car payments on his current salary. Yet these messages were muted because those bodies got hypnotized into believing that justice is paramount. Eventually Jason ended up taking a second job to make both car payments and had to drop out of the project altogether at a time when they needed him most.

Of course, unconditional love and passionately working for a cause are admirable qualities. These stories are not meant to downplay high frequency intentions. They are only to suggest that attention be paid to development of the ego bodies relative to the universal body. In a balanced system, a healthy universal body is a powerful guiding force in life. It gives you the *lived experience* of universal virtues, not imposed ideals. The universal body is inherently inclusive. It does not exclude the ego bodies nor does it entrance them. A hypnotized body is unconscious. The universal body seeks to expand consciousness, not take it away.

The universal and the ego bodies mutually influence each other. When a well-developed universal body is aligned with healthy ego bodies, you have continuity of consciousness on all levels (vital/physical, emotional, mental, universal). You are able to respond to life in a unified manner, without inner conflict. You act as an integrated whole; your ego bodies are infused with unity consciousness. Your life is a reflection of this coherence. You are stable and grounded in the physical world while psycho-emotionally free. You are *in* the world but not *of* it. Your healthy ego bodies are able to carry out the wishes and desires of your universal body, acting in service of unity consciousness. You are able to take your place in the wholeness.

Balanced growth of the universal body starts with a basic hygiene program. To further the proper upbringing of the universal body a development program involves Recognition and Integration.

Universal Body Hygiene

Basic hygiene is a fundamental part of the universal body's nurturance, as this body will blossom when it is attended to and kept clean. Basic hygiene for the universal body starts with assessing the condition of this body through a Mirror Check.

Universal Body Mirror Check

When performing the mirror check you want to pay particular attention to the dimensions and weight of your universal body. Just as good parenting requires careful tracking of an infant's growth, it's important to assess your universal body on an ongoing basis so you can make minor adjustments at the first hint of a problem. If unattended, development of the universal body can get stunted or disproportionate relative to the ego bodies, predisposing you to the Duping and/or Trancing Syndromes described above.

Exercise: Universal Body Mirror Check
Application: At least once a day, to monitor the growth of
your universal body.
Time: 1 minute

- Find a quiet place in which you can focus without
  distraction.

- Take a couple of slow, deep breaths. Close your eyes
  and intentionally shift your attention away from an
  external focus toward an internal focus, awakening
  your internal senses.

- Allow your physical body to relax. Allow your
  emotional body to calm. Allow your mental body to
  clear.

- Visualize a mirror in front of you. Instead of your
  physical body, this mirror is reflecting your universal
  body.

- Notice everything you can about your universal body.
  How does it look today? What color is it? Shape?
  Size? What stands out? Notice the details. Anything
  you need to adjust? Overall condition?

- Whenever this feels complete, open your eyes.

If you find that your universal body is fully developed and
flourishing, compare it with the health of your ego bodies. If it is
disproportionately large relative to your ego bodies, beware of the
Trancing Syndrome. Instead of focusing on the development of
your universal body at this time, go back and revisit the previous
chapters on the vital, emotional and mental bodies, focusing on
their condition and care.

If you find that your universal body is under-developed, compare it with the health of your ego bodies and pay close attention to the Duping Syndrome described above. If duping is at play, the exercises in the remainder of this chapter will help your universal body. If growth is proportionate, and neither duping nor trancing are at play, use the exercises that follow to address developmental needs accordingly.

Be Light

The universal body achieves its full development by working in cooperation with the ego bodies and cannot fully manifest in isolation. However, because Western culture favors the ego bodies, a newly developing universal body can get overly influenced by them and become ego-saturated. The Be Light exercise helps cleanse it of excess ego inergy. The exercise is designed to bring conscious awareness to the universal body and facilitate direct access to its ultra-high frequency inergies. This is accomplished by using your intent to go deeply inside yourself, because doing so increases the frequency. In other words, *in* is *up* in frequency.

Enacting the Be Light exercise on a regular basis helps you access universal inergies and awaken higher-level intuition. The exercise starts with your attention in your heart center so that the quality of love (a high frequency inergy associated with the heart's inergy center) can govern your experience. It also involves filling yourself with light, as light is an archetypal symbol of consciousness. The exercise cannot be rushed; it must be carried out very slowly. Take your time, allowing yourself to be *in* time, not *on* time.

Exercise: Be Light
Application: As needed, to help cleanse the universal body of any ego inergy saturation.
Time: 5-10 minutes

- Find a quiet place in which you can focus without distraction.

- Take a couple of slow, deep breaths. Close your eyes and intentionally shift your attention away from an external focus toward an internal focus, awakening your internal senses.

- Allow your physical body to relax, your emotional body to calm, and your mental body to clear.

- Bring your attention to your heart center.

- Visualize the sun, radiant and bright. Feel the warmth of the sun on your face. Breathe slowly and deeply, filling yourself with the rays of the sun.

- Continue breathing in the light, filling yourself with light . . . until you are completely filled with light. Take your time. Use self-sensing to actually experience this.

- Continue self-sensing and stay with the experience.

- Slowly breathe yourself deeper into your being . . . deeper . . . deeper still.

- Let yourself experience the expansiveness and infinity of consciousness itself. Spend some time here.

- Whenever you are ready, gently breathe yourself back into your physical body. Anchor your awareness in your physical body. Feel your feet on the floor.

- Whenever this feels complete, open your eyes.

Once hygiene is attended to, you can further foster the growth of your universal body with the developmental exercises that follow.

Basic Development

The biggest obstacle to development of the universal body is lack of recognition. This body is oftentimes overlooked while the needs of the other bodies take precedence. The exercises and practices that follow are designed to give the universal body the attention it needs in order to flourish. The development program starts with Recognition.

Recognition

Unity consciousness is the substance of the universal body. However, the universal body needs recognition from you and from your other bodies in order to manifest unity in the material world. The Recognition exercise helps you sustain the primacy of the universal body in your life.

With all the demands of work, family, friends, and personal interests competing for your attention, it's easy to lose focus on the universal body. The following exercise[3] helps keep the universal body in perspective. The triangle is symbolic of your three ego bodies (vital/physical, emotional, and mental) while the yellow color is associated with the intuition aspect of the universal body. This exercise helps bring awareness to your universal body and awaken higher-level intuition.

Exercise: Recognition
Application: As needed, to help you recognize your universal body and to awaken intuition.
Time: 3 minutes

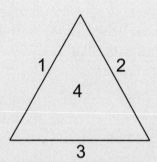

- Find a quiet place in which you can focus without distraction.

- Take a couple of slow, deep breaths. Close your eyes and intentionally shift your attention away from an external focus toward an internal focus, awakening your internal senses.

- Allow your physical body to relax. Allow your emotional body to calm. Allow your mental body to clear.

- Visualize three yellow lines of the same length in front of you and form them into an equilateral triangle (each side is the same length).

- When you feel ready, place your attention on one of the sides of the yellow triangle (position 1). From this position, look over and see the other two sides of the triangle.

- Then when you are ready, move your awareness along the outer periphery of the triangle until you are occupying two of the three sides of the triangle (positions 1 and 2). From this position look over and see the last side of the triangle (position 3).

- When you are ready, move your awareness so you are now occupying all three sides of the triangle and looking into the center (position 4).

- Then when you are ready, move yourself into the center of the yellow triangle (position 4). Notice that from this position you can see all three sides of the triangle and beyond.

- In this visualization the three sides of the triangle represent your physical, emotional, and mental bodies while the center position represents your universal body.

- From your position in the center, remind yourself that you have a physical body but you are not your physical body—you are more than that. You feed your physical body and care for it but you are not this body.

- You have an emotional body and so you experience feelings. Sometimes you feel happy, sad, irritated, angry or afraid, but you are not your emotions. You are much more than that.

- You have a mental body. You think thoughts, analyze ideas, and figure things out, but you are not your intellect. You are much more than that.

- You are a pure inergy center, a center of consciousness, a center of will, capable of directing your physical body, emotions and thoughts to manifest what you will.

- Whenever this feels complete, you can open your eyes.

Integration

Your universal body needs the cooperation of the other bodies in order to manifest unity consciousness in the material world. However, oftentimes the other bodies have agendas of their own and do not want to integrate with the universal body. The Integration exercise[4] is designed to align the lower frequency bodies with the higher inergies of the universal body. Again, the metaphor of light is used to symbolize consciousness.

Exercise: Integration
Application: As needed, to help your ego bodies recognize your universal body.
Time: 6 minutes

- Find a quiet place in which you can focus without distraction.

- Take a couple of slow, deep breaths. Close your eyes and intentionally shift your attention away from an external focus toward an internal focus, awakening your internal senses.

- Allow your physical body to relax. Allow your emotional body to calm. Allow your mental body to clear.

- Focus your attention in your heart. Notice that you have a flame burning in your heart. Clearly visualize the flame.

- Notice how, when you breathe in, the flame grows brighter and stronger. When you breathe out the flame grows more radiant.

- Keep breathing, gently and deeply, allowing the flame to grow, breathing in the light, filling yourself with the light . . . until you become the light.

- Then visualize your three ego bodies standing in front of you (physical, emotional, and mental).

- Your physical body is the first one to notice you. It becomes aware of the body of light that you are and agrees to let go of its way of doing things in order to follow the light.

- See your physical body indicate its agreement to you in some way (maybe it nods, smiles, or says it agrees). Then it stands off to the side.

- Next, your emotional body becomes aware of the body of light that you are. It agrees to give up its desires and impulses in order to follow the light.

- See your emotional body signal its agreement in some way and then stand off to the side with your physical body.

- Next, your mental body becomes aware of the body of light that you are and it agrees to let go of its opinions, of wanting to figure it out and be right, in order to follow the light.

- See your mental body signal its agreement in some way and then stand with the emotional and physical bodies.

- Next, visualize your three ego bodies melting together to form one body. Then this body unites with the body of light and they fuse into one integrated body. Hold this image for as long as you'd like.

- Whenever this feels complete, open your eyes.

The universal body is recognized and sustained by keeping the ego bodies aligned with it as much as possible.

Meta-Conscious

Further development of the universal body involves working directly with the consciousness continuum, all of it—from selective awareness, individual consciousness, the collective, and intuitive, to unity consciousness. Supportive practices involve using consciousness to become more aware of itself. In other words, to keep attention focused on consciousness, to be meta-conscious (*meta* meaning *beyond* or *self-referential*).

The meta-conscious exercise has three phases. The first phase is to become conscious of your individual awareness, specifically the selection aspect of it. Phase 2 involves making different choices about where you place your attention, when applicable. The third phase is designed to recalibrate your individual consciousness to a higher frequency. Because consciousness is omnipresent, these are not so much exercises as ongoing practices.

- **Phase 1** addresses the selection aspect

- **Phase 2** addresses making necessary adjustments to the selection aspect

- **Phase 3** addresses your overall individual con-sciousness structure

Phase 1

In the first phase, the goal is to reclaim your selection process by paying attention to what you pay attention to. It involves heightening awareness through self-observation. There is no need to change anything. You want to do your best to stay aware of what you focus your attention on in any given moment. Sometimes this practice is called *mindfulness*.

Since tracking every waking moment of your awareness would be a daunting task, it's helpful to make incremental observations. Depending on your current level of awareness, you may want to draw attention to your attention, say, every hour or two. It's also helpful to keep a journal and make notes. Your journal entries may look something like this:

Sample: Meta-Conscious Phase 1

7-8 a.m.   Got ready for the day and thought about a challenging interaction with a friend

8-9 a.m.   Worked on a proposal, some defensive thoughts and blaming friend thoughts

9-10 a.m.   Returned phone calls, brightened the day for several people, more proposal writing

10-11 a.m.   Surfed the web, got distracted by headlines and reading about torture (very depressing), some sensationalized movie star stories, back on track to research zero-point energy, very enlightening

11-12 p.m.   Remembered a dream, analyzed it, then focused on writing the proposal

12-1 p.m.   Lunch with a friend, fun but lots of talk criticizing local politics

1-2 p.m.   Ran a few errands, got overwhelmed by the crowded stores

2-3 p.m.   Did online banking, web-surfing, more reading of sensationalized headlines and stories

3-4 p.m.   Focused on proposal writing, distracted by phone calls, I was terse

4-5 p.m.   Proposal writing, stayed focused and productive

5-6 p.m.   Proposal writing, stayed mostly focused

6-7 p.m.   Food prep and eating, enjoyed a delicious meal

7-8 p.m.   Eating and cleaning up, back to thinking of friend, sad now

8-9 p.m.   Watched a movie that was mostly confusing and somewhat violent

9-10 p.m.   More of the movie watching

10-11 p.m.   Got ready for bed still trying to figure out that movie, a bit troubling

Establishing a clear intent in the morning to stay aware throughout the day and setting reminders is very helpful. Again, the goal of this phase is simply to observe: to become more aware of where you place your awareness. This phase can take about 1-3 weeks, enough time to establish a baseline of your attention domain. Once you are more aware of the focus of your attention, you can make choices accordingly.

Practice: Meta-Conscious Phase 1
Supplies: Notebook or journal to make notes
Application: To help expand consciousness by bringing awareness to what you pay attention to.
Time: Ongoing for about 1-3 weeks

- Start your day by setting a clear intent to notice what you pay attention to.

- Pick a specific time increment to check-in and keep a log.

- Throughout your day do your best to stay aware of where you place your attention, what you select to pay attention to.

- Make notes in your journal to track your awareness.

Phase 2

The second phase invites you to review your selection process and make any indicated changes. With Phase 2, you are asked to shift to higher frequency inergy input (those aligned with unity consciousness) when possible. Whatever you focus attention on you bring inergy to, so your attention is a kind of inergy currency. It's best to be conscious of where you are investing your inergy currency. This phase serves to eradicate any lower frequency, separative inputs. It is accomplished by reviewing the results of Phase 1 with an overlay of low versus high frequency inergies. How much of your attention is focused on sensory input that evokes separateness (guilt, fear, disdain, pride, etc.) and how much on unity (willingness, neutrality, acceptance, peace, etc.)? To help with the exercise, here is a review of the inergy calibrations of various states of consciousness from Chapter 9:[5]

High Frequency States

Level	Calibration
Peace	600
Love	500

Reason	400
Acceptance	350
Willingness	310
Neutrality	250

Low Frequency States

Level	Calibration
Pride	175
Desire	125
Fear	100
Grief	75
Apathy	50
Guilt	30

From the journal excerpt above, a consciousness-centered review indicates the following:

Low Frequency: friend blame; torture/depressing; movie star/gossip; criticizing local politics; terse phone call; sad about friend; violent/confusing movie

High Frequency: uplifted people; enlightening zero-point research; insightful dream-analysis; fun with friend; enjoyed meal; productive proposal writing

Given these results I would make the following adjustments to what I choose to pay attention to: stop the blame and sadness about the friend, stop reading about torture and movie stars, stop criticizing local politics, stop watching violent movies. Replace these activities with higher-calibrated choices. Do the mental body Perspective exercise from Chapter 9 with regard to the friend situation and the local politicians.

After a period of time Phase 1 may be discontinued and Phase 2 ideally becomes more of a way of life.

Practice: Meta-Conscious Phase 2
Application: To help nurture the universal body by
paying attention to what you pay attention to and
then consciously choosing higher frequency input.
Time: Ongoing

- Review your journal from Phase I to determine
  how much of your awareness is focused on lower
  frequencies and how much on higher.

- Make adjustments accordingly.

- Throughout the day whenever you find that you are
  paying attention to lower frequency inergies do your
  best to shift your focus to something of a higher
  calibration.

Phase 2 asks you to consciously choose higher frequency
input. It is concerned with the selection aspect of your awareness.
Phase 3 highlights your individual consciousness structure: what
state of consciousness do you bring to any given situation?

Phase 3

We are all united by consciousness. Consciousness is the
great mediator between the ego and the universal bodies—between
individuality and unity. In this respect, your thoughts are not your
own; your feelings are not your own. Even your awareness is not
your own! Your personal actions, thoughts, feelings and awareness
are directly impacting others via the universal body. We are,
therefore, called upon to act with conscience, to be responsible for
our participation in the continuum of consciousness. The moral
imperative of unity consciousness mandates us to take responsibility
for what we contribute to and take from the consciousness matrix.

This phase of the Meta-Conscious exercise is meant to recalibrate your individual consciousness to a higher frequency, aligning it more with unity.

With the Phase 3 practice, you are asked to notice what state of consciousness you bring to any situation and to shift to higher frequency states in the moment. Every moment is an opportunity to expand individual awareness to unity consciousness. Shifting to a higher frequency state of mind may sound like denial or even rationalization, harkening back to the Duping and Trancing Syndromes. But there is a crucial difference: this practice involves the expansion of consciousness whereas denial and rationalization do not. Let's look at examples of each.

Say you have an important outing planned for the day. You wake up in the morning, throw open the blinds, and see a dark sky full of rain clouds. You feel disappointed and a bit anxious. If you are in denial you will think, "What a nice sunny day!" As the word implies, you will deny the existence of the clouds, pretend you don't see them, and instead substitute a positive picture. Denial shrinks consciousness by excluding aspects of reality. Whatever you don't want to see, you simply deny exists. This may be fairly innocuous when it comes to clouds in the sky. However, denial can be more detrimental if it is applied to other things, like that strange growth on your arm that you don't want to deal with, or your loved one's drinking problem.

As for the second trap, if you are rationalizing you will throw open the blinds, see the dark clouds, feel disappointed or anxious and say to yourself, "Well, the clouds are a good thing because we need some rain anyway and when I go out today I won't have to worry about getting sunburned." You will think up all the reasons you can to justify why the clouds are good, using your mental body to put a positive spin on the situation. Rationalization is an indulgence of the mental body. It deprives the universal body of growth and shrinks consciousness by redirecting awareness to a false reality. Rationalization creates a false reality by painting happy faces on situations that mask the underlying truth. That strange growth on your arm is actually cute and helps to distract people from noticing your dark arm hair. Your loved one's drinking is a good way for him to bond with his friends and co-workers and get ahead in the company. The real issues are not dealt with because the rationalization becomes the reality.

If, instead, you are engaged in Meta-Conscious practice to support the growth of your universal body, you will see the dark clouds, register any disappointment or anxiety from your emotional body, and understand this for what it is: an emotional body reaction, nothing more, nothing less. Your emotional body, with its forces of attraction and repulsion, does not want the clouds to be there so it inergetically repulses them, which causes separation. Consciousness to the rescue! As the great unifying force, consciousness can mend the separation.

You stretch your consciousness to connect with the clouds, so to speak. Instead of denying them or trying to change them you accept them. You perceive them as they are, without judgment or blame. You don't make them wrong or bad, nor do you make them right or good. They simply are. You are at peace with them. You connect your awareness with the clouds as they are and appreciate that the day is perfect for you as it is. No need to deny reality, no need to put a positive spin on it. It is what it is. You are neutral.

There is a tendency to regard ultra-high frequency states such as acceptance, neutrality, or peace, as being weak, as if once you achieve such a state you will cease to act in the world, become complacent and ineffectual. This is not the case. Actions continue to happen, they just have a different inergy behind them. You still bring your rain jacket and umbrella for the outing. You see the growth on your arm for what it is and are willing to deal with it accordingly. You see your loved one's alcohol consumption for what it is and are willing to address it. You are not acting out of fear or anger or any other lower frequency inergy. You accept the situation. That state of acceptance, as an ultra-high inergy, has a calming influence on your emotional and mental bodies and allows you the freedom to act in the best possible way.

The Phase 3 practice invites you to recalibrate your individual consciousness structure to align with unity consciousness (and other ultra-high frequency inergies) as much as possible. Doing a review in the evening to track your progress is helpful.

Practice: Meta-Conscious Phase 3
Application: To nurture the universal body by becoming aware of what state of consciousness you bring to any situation and intentionally choosing states more aligned with unity.
Time: Ongoing

- Throughout the day whenever you find that you are in a lower frequency inergy state, do your best to shift your consciousness to a higher calibration, more aligned with unity (i.e., neutrality, acceptance, willingness, peace).

- Avoid falling into the traps of denial or rationalization.

- Do an evening review of your day to identify successes and places where there is room for improvement. Make notes in your journal as needed.

The meta-conscious practices help your universal body grow by bringing awareness to consciousness, thereby expanding it. In addition, development of the universal body requires unity-in-action in the world.

Unity Action

Since unity consciousness comprises the substance of the universal body, validation of this body includes affirming the interconnectedness of all through action in the world. The exercise[6] below invites you to serve unity consciousness in a tangible way by doing something good for someone every day. Planning what you are going to do as an intentional, purposeful action has substantial inergy mobilized behind it. Keep a journal where you record your plan for the day. Then check in the evening to review how well you carried it out. Instead of waiting for an opportunity, actively create an opportunity to help.

Here is a reminder from Chapter 7 of how intent works best: *be sure your good deed is aligned with what the person wants and not just what you want for the person.* The primary purpose of the deed is to validate unity, to affirm connection with the person. This cannot happen if you impose your will on someone, opposing theirs. Say your son doesn't like to eat breakfast but you think breakfast is important, so your good deed is to prepare a fabulous breakfast for him. This does not qualify as a Unity Action. Check your intent. Ask yourself if you are motivated by what your son wants for himself or by what you want for him. Choose something that you know brings him joy. Remove an obstacle from his life, create an opening, help him flourish, or inspire him on his path. You increase your inergy if you use it in the right way, in service of unity. When you are tapped-in to the collective and acting in alignment with it, you will be carried by its inergy. You may have heard it said, to those who give it will be given.

Another word of caution: *be sure your good deed is aligned with what you want as well.* Say your employee loves Gangsta Rap music but you won't allow her to play it at work because the sound waves travel through the walls to your office and you don't like it. Your plan for a Unity Action is to let her play her favorite music for a week. A deed that brings the other person joy but goes against what you want does not qualify as a Unity Action either. Instead, it's better to find something that agrees with both of you. This will affirm inergetic connectedness.

Exercise: Unity Action
Supplies: A journal or notebook to make notes
Application: To validate unity by intentionally and
consistently helping others.
Time: Varies

- Plan to do something good for someone the next day. Make note of who it is, what you will do, and how you will do it.

- Check your intent. Make sure the deed is aligned with what the person wants and what you want so as to affirm unity.

- Carry out your plan.

- In the evening, review what you did, how well you did it, and how it was received.

- If a day passes in which you have not helped someone in the flesh, so to speak, give them the support through visualization, as this validates unity consciousness on the internal levels and helps create the inergy pathways for improvements to happen.

- The same guidelines as above apply: help in a way that agrees with both of you.

- Visualize someone in need of help.

- Then see yourself giving the person what is needed. Dramatize it as much as possible.

As mentioned in the previous chapter, unity is an appealing concept when it comes to feeling connected with the people and things we like. However, unity also requires connecting with those we don't like, as there is no separation. This necessitates connection *especially* with those we do not like. The next exercise is designed to facilitate this.

Inergy Mends

There is a strong tendency to identify with people who hold the same views as we do and to inergetically separate (through thoughts, feelings or actions) from those who don't. This is a mistake, as it perpetuates separation, which is contrary to reality. A typical example is to believe in peace yet hate those who advocate war. This is inergetically incoherent. In this instance, the ego bodies are actually resonant with the inergy of hate. We may talk about peace but we are not truly aligned with it. We are inergetically broadcasting hate to the collective consciousness, and therefore actively perpetuating war, the very thing we profess to be trying to stop. A healthy universal body requires acknowledgment of essential oneness in thoughts, words, and deeds.

The peaceful kingdom of Tibet in Southeast Asia was invaded by the Chinese in 1950. By 1959 tens of thousands of Tibetans had been killed and the Tibetan leader, the fourteenth Dalai Lama, was exiled to India. Destruction of Tibetan cultural icons, buildings, religious artifacts, and language took place. Key members of the international community condemned the violent invasion by the Chinese, but to no avail. After living in exile from his home for almost 50 years, the Dalai Lama was recently asked to support the use of economic sanctions against China to help facilitate a peaceful resolution to the illegal occupation of his homeland. His response was that he could not support such action because it would harm the Chinese and he did not want to do that. In a poignant example of unity consciousness, the Dalai Lama showed us that *the one who enacts harm is in greater need of love than the one who has been harmed.*

In the exercise that follows you are asked to reconnect with someone (or a group) with whom you have inergetically separated. This could be someone you don't like, someone who has done you wrong, or someone you don't get along with. The exercise asks you to invoke the palpable sensation of love. If you don't have easy access to this inergy, you may need to visualize situations that conjure it up, say, images of a newborn baby, memories of your wedding day, thinking of favorite loved ones, experiences of universal love, any instances that evoke love. You are then asked to transfer that love to your chosen person (or group). Once again, the exercise focuses attention in your heart center (love) and uses the metaphor of light (consciousness).

Do your best to extend a general attitude of compassion to others, loving the other as yourself. If you slip and relapse into separatism, do this exercise as quickly as possible to inergetically mend the situation.

Exercise: Inergy Mends
Application: As needed, to affirm unity inergetically by reconnecting as quickly as possible with someone from whom you have disconnected.
Time: 5 minutes

- Find a quiet place in which you can focus without distraction.

- Take a couple of slow, deep breaths. Close your eyes and intentionally shift your attention away from an external focus toward an internal focus, awakening your internal senses.

- Allow your physical body to relax. Allow your emotional body to calm. Allow your mental body to clear.

- Focus your attention in your heart. Access the inergy of love. If it is not available on command, visualize situations that invoke love inside you.

- When the feeling of love is tangible and strong, visualize the person you do not like. See them bathed in light, with light all around them.

- Send the person your love and visualize them smiling and receiving your love.

- Hold this for about 1 minute.

- When you are ready open your eyes.

- The next time you see this person or think of them, do your best to remember love and to increase your love for them.

Helping the universal body to develop and advancing unity consciousness means staying in the inergy of connectedness even when faced with situations we don't like.

Advanced Techniques

So far we have addressed practices that validate the universal body through connection with others. But sometimes it happens that we, ourselves, are in need of inergetic support from the universal level. This calls for advanced techniques.

Cosmos

In the previous chapter we discussed the Elastic Effect, how consciousness expands and contracts depending on how you use it. If you hyper-focus your awareness on something or someone, your consciousness (and your universal body) will shrink accordingly. Sometimes we can get stuck in a contracted state and have a hard time finding our way out. Each of the bodies has an agenda of its own and can pull us in different directions. If your awareness gets locked onto one of your bodies and/or onto a problem you are dealing with, it becomes very difficult to resolve.

You can observe events from the standpoint of your ego bodies or that of your universal body. Although the perspective of the ego bodies is limited, the tendency is to gravitate to that limited viewpoint. The higher frequency range of the universal body affords a much broader view, with more degrees of freedom, and includes the ego bodies. Nothing is left out. Along with the power of expanded observation comes choice: freedom of choice. The exercise[7] that follows expands the universal body and is useful if you find your awareness is too tightly focused, especially in dealing with a challenging situation.

Exercise: Cosmos
Application: As needed, to help expand a contracted consciousness structure; to utilize the freedom and perspective gained from identifying with your universal body.
Time: 8-10 minutes

- Find a quiet place in which you can focus without distraction.

- Take a couple of slow, deep breaths. Close your eyes and intentionally shift your attention away from an external focus toward an internal focus, awakening your internal senses.

- Allow your physical body to relax. Allow your emotional body to calm. Allow your mental body to clear.

- Call to mind your favorite peaceful place in nature that has grass, trees, and open sky. Visualize yourself there.

- Self-sense and feel the warmth of the sun on your face. Breathe slowly and deeply, filling yourself with the rays of the sun.

- Let the peace of the surroundings penetrate your whole being. Sense the peace. Take your time with this step.

- Let your consciousness expand, dissolving any boundaries, so that you become one with the grass and the trees.

- Become one with the breeze and the light.

- Become one with the sky above.

- Think about the great space beyond our galaxy.

- Project your awareness to a planet far away.

- Imagine that you are sitting on a planet in a far off galaxy looking through limitless space at planet Earth where you exist.

- See the planet Earth below you.

- Think of who you are and what you are compared to infinite space.

- You can stay in this state for as long as you like. Spend at least 1 minute here.

- Whenever you are ready gently breathe yourself back to planet Earth, back to your location, back into your physical body. Feel the ground beneath you. Anchor your awareness in your physical body.

- Whenever this feels complete, open your eyes.

Once Cosmos mode is established you can use the expanded state of consciousness to observe aspects of your ego bodies that might otherwise be invisible.

Inside-Out

In the previous chapter we discussed how unity means being one with everything—the flowers, the trees, the breeze, as well as those things we don't like—the irritating neighbor, the demanding boss, the serial killer, the terrorist. The problems of the world did not arise out in the world, outside of us. They are problems inside us. If they show up out in the world, they already exist inside of us, in our consciousness.

In looking at the world situation it's easy to see complex problems and feel powerless to do anything to make a difference. The following exercise gives a way to help by cleaning up the consciousness structure from which the problems originate. Consciousness is primary: if it shows up outside, it already exists inside. Consciousness is the mediating force between the internal and the external, between the individual and the collective. As in the Hundredth Monkey effect, when you do your part to transform your individual consciousness, you help to uplift all of humanity. The Inside-Out exercise invites you to use your perception of problems in the external world to reciprocally identify and clean out those very issues in your internal consciousness structure. Let's look more closely at how this might be done.

In the aftermath of the World Trade Center devastation when terrorism took center stage in the public eye, members of an Inner Clarity (IC)[8] group I was hosting at the time took the opportunity to cleanse ourselves of internal terrorism. To be sure, no one in the group had the slightest inclination to commit acts of terrorism against anyone. However, upon deeper inquiry we discovered similar inergies lodged away inside each of us. These took various forms.

The IC group adopted a typical definition of terrorism as the starting point: the use of violence or threats to intimidate, coerce, or induce a state of fear or submission. One woman discovered that she kept her boyfriend under threat of leaving him. She had carried out her plan once in the past and he was devastated. After they reunited, when conflict arose, she took to reminding him that she would leave again since he wasn't giving her what she wanted. This was enough to frighten him into submission. Another woman realized that she was "terrorizing" her son by threatening to take his cherished cell phone if he disobeyed her. Another found that she was "terrorizing" herself by having convinced herself that she would gain weight every time she put something in her mouth. This kept her in a constant fear of food. She only half jokingly noted the dire symbolism of being "blown up" by the terrorizing food.

The revelations of the IC group may seem frivolous and hyper-inflated. Of course, there are ways to pay attention to food intake, remove a youngster's cell phone, and talk about ending a relationship that have nothing to do with terrorism, and can be quite the opposite. Discerning the inergetic origins of your actions is an inside job. However, if the inergetic trace is there, from the perspective of consciousness, those inergy impulses and their accompanying thought-forms, left unchecked, eventually precipitate out into denser manifestations. They do not start nor will they end on the physical level. They represent specific states of consciousness. Identifying and transforming such underlying core states is profoundly life altering, not only for the individual but also for the collective. If we want to change the world, we must change our consciousness because consciousness is primary. There is no separation, only unity.

To be clear, this "inside-out" approach to dealing with issues is not meant to replace conscientious action in the world. It is meant to address the behind-the-scenes inergy aspects of an issue. Any issue can potentially be used in this way as a change-agent at the level of consciousness. *If it shows up outside it already exists inside.* The IC group also worked on pollution, greed, and war. In doing the exercise, the issue is not to be taken literally but understood inergetically, or symbolically. You want to get in touch with the quality of the inergy behind the issue and locate it within yourself, to the best of your ability. This demands a high degree of self-observation, a required faculty in this advanced training level.

We found there is a direct correlation between the volatility of the external issue and the level of internal identification with the issue. In other words, the more emotionally charged an issue, the more there is to clean. You resonate most with external issues that mirror your internal consciousness (remember the tuning fork metaphor from Chapter 5). This applies to world issues as well as qualities we see in other people. You may first see the issue externally, as a social issue, or as a problem in another person. But if you have an emotional charge about it, chances are you have your own version of it running inside you. As one member of the IC group was fond of saying, "If you spot it, you got it!"

The exercise below invites you to identify a topic or issue that has a particular emotional charge before you begin. Pick a problem that you want to explore with the intent of changing it internally, at the level of consciousness. In Stage 1 of the exercise, you are asked to engage your conceptual mind and assume Director's Mode to self-observe your bodies and locate any inergies resonant with the chosen topic. Do your best to understand the inergy behind the issue. Be careful not to interpret the issue literally. Once the underlying resonant core-states are revealed, the second stage of the exercise[9] contains a way to use the light and power of consciousness to transform them.

Exercise: Inside-Out
Application: As needed, to help make a difference
in the world by using negative external issues to
clean out internal resonant inergies.
Time: Varies

- Find a quiet place in which you can focus without distraction.

- Take a couple of slow, deep breaths. Close your eyes and intentionally shift your attention away from an external focus toward an internal focus, awakening your internal senses.

- Allow your physical body to relax. Allow your emotional body to calm. Allow your mental body to clear.

- Use your intent to connect with your conceptual mind and activate Director's Mode.

- Call to mind your chosen issue.

- **Stage 1**: Self-observe to discover your version of the issue. Examine each of your ego bodies thoroughly, looking for any hint of the issue, the inergy behind the issue, or related topics. Find as many resonant inergies as possible. Observe how your version of this issue plays out in your life. Look deeply and carefully. Take your time. Be thorough.

- When this is complete, you are ready for Stage 2.

- **Stage 2**: Visualize a searchlight of potentially great brilliance and intensity on your forehead, but the light is not yet projecting outward. Your mind is held steady in the light.

- Recognize the issue you wish to transform without feeding it any new inergy (i.e., you can visualize it as an image, hear it as a word, see it as a picture, sense it, or feel it).

- Consciously activate the power of your intent. Turn on the searchlight on your forehead, and see a vivid beam of light stream forth and contact the issue. Visualize a broad, brilliant beam, pouring forth from your illumined mind.

- Say to yourself (self-talk with great conviction):

  - "The power of the light prevents the appearance of (the issue)."

  - "The power of the light neutralizes the inergy behind the issue."

- Visualize the following in succession:

  - That the light makes a definite impact upon the issue.

  - That the issue is being absorbed by the light.

  - That the light fully dissipates the issue.

- Then withdraw your beam of light and anchor your awareness in the center of your head.

This exercise is a service activity. In a two-way process, you shape the collective consciousness and, in turn, are shaped by it. The exercises in this chapter provide a way of raising the frequency of your individual consciousness to help develop your universal body and do your part in service of the whole.

All is interconnected via the universal body. Thus, you are called upon to pay attention to what you contribute to and take from the collective consciousness in your individual, moment-to-moment, day-to-day life and do your best to actualize unity on all levels. The goal is to expand consciousness, to connect the dots of your experience, to increase your individual awareness to the extent that you perceive the interconnectedness of all in each and every moment—everything all together, all at once, here and now—and act from that awareness.

> As you work with your own inergy
> Any expansion of consciousness you may achieve
> No matter how small it may seem to be
> Helps to uplift all of humanity.

Chapter Eleven

Endless Energy

At the start of this book we discussed how everything is energy, vibrating at different frequencies. We discussed how this energy is intimately coupled with information, which we call inergy, and that you are comprised of four main inergy bodies. These inergy bodies are responsible for your overall energy levels. Your vital body, in particular, plays a key role in supplying your vitality, your "get-up-and-go" energy. However, because your vital body interfaces with your emotional, mental, and universal bodies, all of your bodies impact your energy levels. We've explored these bodies individually and now it's time to put them back together and look at your inergy system as a whole. We'll discover ways to access higher-level guidance, gain inergy assistance in decision-making, and learn how inergy moves within your multidimensional system.

Your inergy bodies exist on a continuum ranging from low to high frequencies, which means you have the equipment to process four distinct levels of experience simultaneously: sensation (through your vital/physical body), emotion (through your emotional body), thought (through your mental body) and consciousness (through your universal body). Your four inergy bodies are the "vehicles of experience" that make this possible. If you are not using all four channels of experience to the fullest you are limiting yourself. The fact that we occupy these four levels of existence makes us quite complex. The very nature of our multidimensional inergy system means it's easy to feel conflicted inside. Each body has an agenda of its own that can pull us in different directions. The key is to identify which body (or bodies) is getting in the way, do interventions to help it, and align with the universal body as much as possible. We have one last exercise that is designed to assist with this.

Inergy Guidance

You've probably experienced times in your life when you needed to make an important decision and felt confused about what to do. You likely have also experienced a desire to move forward in a particular direction in your life but found it difficult, as if invisible forces were working against you. These challenges are apt to happen if your inergy bodies are not aligned. This exercise helps you discover how your bodies are influencing you and is useful in accessing guidance from your universal body.

In the exercise you are asked to place four empty chairs side by side. If you don't have access to four chairs you can substitute four pillows, or even four sheets of paper placed on the floor on which you can stand or sit. Position the chairs side by side with enough room so you can sit in each chair and move from one to the next. The four positions are meant to represent your four bodies—1) physical, 2) emotional, 3) mental, and 4) universal—in sequential order. You are asked to sit in each chair and speak from the perspective of the appropriate body, allowing each body to have its say and weigh-in on the issue. You may want a notebook to jot down your responses.

Exercise: Inergy Guidance
Supplies: Notebook to make notes, four chairs
Setup: In a quiet place in which you can focus
without distraction, position the four chairs side by side
so you can take turns sitting in each one.

Application: As needed, to help identify which inergy body is out of alignment and/or to get in touch with higher frequency guidance.
Time: 15 minutes

- Standing near where you have positioned the four chairs, take a couple of deep breaths. Close your eyes and intentionally shift your attention away from an external focus toward an internal focus, awakening your internal senses.

- Allow your physical body to relax. Allow your emotional body to calm. Allow your mental body to clear.

- Focus your intent on attaining responses that are in the highest good. Then clearly pose the question that you're seeking guidance for (i.e., Should I move to New York?) or state the issue that you feel blocked around (i.e., I want a new career).

- Sit in the first chair, which is meant to represent your physical body. Use your intent to focus your attention exclusively on your physical body, to the best of your ability. Shift into Director's Mode and ask your physical body the question.

- Then allow your physical body to give its input regarding the issue. Allow it to speak through you and voice its concerns, wishes, wants and desires about the topic. Make notes in your notebook if you wish.

- When this feels complete, move into the next chair. This chair is meant to represent your emotional body. Sitting in the emotional body chair, use your intent to focus your attention exclusively on your emotional body. Shift into Director's Mode and ask your emotional body the question.

- Then allow your emotional body to give its input regarding the issue. Allow it to speak through you and voice its concerns, wishes, wants and desires about the topic. Make notes in your notebook.

- Repeat this step with your mental and universal bodies, one at a time, moving into each representative chair, allowing each body to have its say. Make notes as necessary along the way.

- When you have finished, review your notes to see which body or bodies are not aligned with your statement. To receive higher frequency guidance pay particular attention to what your universal body has to say in response to your question or statement.

The Inergy Guidance exercise can help you sort through the internal influences of your inergy bodies and clarify what you really want. It can also help refine your wants and aspirations by opening up a focused channel of communication with your universal body.

Go a Step Higher

Einstein once said that a problem cannot be solved on the level at which it was created. This provides an important clue when it comes to situations that don't seem to respond to same-level treatments. To be clear, same-level interventions (i.e., trying to solve a physical body problem on the physical level) can be necessary and helpful, but they don't always work. In these situations, going to the next higher level of complexity often holds the key.

Your bodies work together to the extent that to change one body is to change them all. But the inergy travels through the bodies in a particular way—from higher frequency to lower. To get a better idea of this, think of a household heating system. It consists of several components—output ducts in each room, the furnace itself, the electricity that powers the furnace, and a thermostat. Each of these components is distinct, yet vital to the operation of the system and each component represents a level of complexity. The ducts are at the most basic level. The furnace is more complex. The electricity even more so. Finally, the thermostat represents the highest level of complexity because it controls everything. The thermostat determines the functioning of the entire system. It unites the components to operate as a whole. The thermostat is at the highest level of complexity but that does not make it more important than the furnace, electricity, or ducts.

Similarly, your inergy system contains several components (your ego bodies) that are united together into a coordinated whole by your universal body (consciousness). The universal body, like the thermostat, is at the highest level of complexity but it needs your other bodies in order to function. The universal body has more components under its control. When changes are made further up the level of complexity, those changes affect the lower levels more dramatically. However, when it comes to conventional approaches to health, there is a bottom-up focus: every ailment, no matter which body is involved, is addressed by altering the functioning of the dense physical (lowest frequency) body. We are told that surgeries and medications will help the physical body and that physically altering the brain's chemistry is the way to feel better emotionally and think more clearly. But there is little focus on how the higher bodies affect the lower. In fact, they do so to a much larger degree.

The implications are thus: if your physical body is misbehaving, look into the functioning of your vital body to help resolve it. If you are having problems with vitality, examine your emotional body. If there is an emotional body issue, the mental body holds the key. With a mental body concern, turn to the universal body to help. Going to the next higher level of complexity means bringing in faster-frequency inergies to assist. This approach is not meant to replace caring for the body that is in need. It's simply a way to enhance those efforts, especially when such efforts produce limited results. The physical body alone cannot address all the needs of the multidimensional bodies. Intervening at a higher level of complexity is often more efficient. Ultimately, the lower frequency bodies must respond to the higher, just as the furnace responds to the command of the thermostat.

The Recalibration Effect

If you make a change in frequency at the universal level it will cause a change in the mental body. If you shift something at the mental level it will impact the emotional, and so forth. The higher level the change, the more impact it will have on the lower bodies. This can take two forms. One is that your lower bodies easily adjust to the higher frequency and function better immediately. This is the most desirable outcome and is usually the case. The intent of this book is to create high functioning inergy health. However, through the process of recalibrating, sometimes it happens that your lower bodies react to the higher frequency by becoming temporarily dysfunctional as they adjust to the changes.

This Recalibration Effect shows up most vividly on the physical level because that level is the most dense. Let's say you gain insight into a situation that results in a sudden shift, a consciousness expanding "a-ha" realization, or maybe you transform a low frequency repetitive thought-pattern into higher frequency thought-forms. If the change is particularly potent, it may "cascade down" or "precipitate-out" in your lower bodies and translate into some kind of physical symptom. This could result in temporary fatigue or even manifest as a physical ailment such as a headache, sore throat, sinus congestion, or indigestion. The effect depends on your vital body's unique way of expressing through your physical layer. Sometimes this is called a *healing reaction* or *healing crisis*.

It refers to physical symptoms caused by inergy changes in your system that are expressing out through your physical body.

The bottom line is that unpleasant physical expressions are not always bad. Sometimes they are a good indicator of inergy changes happening on other levels and are best understood this way. There is a tendency to identify the physical layer as the exclusive indicator of wellbeing when it's not. We do this at the expense of the other bodies. The slightest physical malady is seen as something wrong and we want to stop it immediately. We take medications, herbs and supplements to treat the symptom. Inergetically speaking, this can have the effect of closing off a channel of expression. To be clear, I am not advocating that you empty out your medicine cabinet and throw everything away. I am inviting you to become aware of your inergy system as a whole so you can identify when the Recalibration Effect may be at play.

When recalibration is happening, the inergy moves through your system in such a way that it needs to express out through your physical layer. In these instances, physical symptoms are an affirmation of changes in the inergy bodies. If inergy channels of expression are artificially closed off through chemical interventions in the physical body, the inergy must find another avenue of expression. This can result in a different set of symptoms physically, or in another body. You can get rid of the scratchy throat but end up with a backache, or worse. If channels of expression continue to be artificially closed off, the inergy is not allowed to express out and can become trapped in your system, potentially causing deeper and more severe imbalances.

The solution is simple but not easy. That is, allow the small symptoms to play out. Instead of taking a cough-suppressant, spend the day in bed resting. This is easier said than done, I know. However, if you want to be inergy healthy, you must pay attention to your inergy bodies. Giving them a break from constant stimulation through periods of quiet inactivity, silence, and downtime allows them to recover. *Your inergy system is a highly complex and intelligent system.* Left to its own devices, it is extremely resilient.

It will strive to right itself and return to balance on its own and may do this much more readily when unencumbered by artificial interventions.

An important key to identifying the Recalibration Effect is to stay in touch with your inergy bodies on an ongoing basis. This can be accomplished by devoting just a few minutes each day to the Mirror Check exercises included in this book. The Recalibration Effect is characterized by feeling good on the inside but not so good on the outside. In other words, your inergy bodies are doing well but your physical body is expressing some symptom. If this is the case, chances are an inergy shift has happened at the higher levels and is vibrating out through your system. Because it is comprised of dense inergy, your physical body feels the effects of high frequency shifts the most. It is the stage where the dynamic interactions of your inergy bodies play out most vividly.

Endless Energy

This book is about dynamic interactions. It's about human energy—where it comes from, how it works, and how to have more of it consistently. It takes the new science of energy medicine, translates it into clear and simple terms, then spells out essential ways for maintaining energy health.

I have enjoyed being your energy health guide and trust the program outlined in the book has been beneficial for you. But, of course, the training doesn't end here. Hopefully *Endless Energy* will stay at your fingertips as your new Home Health Guide for the 21st Century. May endless energy be yours forever.

Everything is energy . . .
You are energy . . .
You are everything . . .
Energy can neither be created nor destroyed . . .
You can neither be created nor destroyed . . .

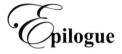
Epilogue

Before and After

At the start of the book (Chapter 2) I described each of the four bodies and included exercises to help you attain robust inergy health. After learning about your inergy constitution and practicing the exercises you may want to repeat the inergy body inventory for "before and after" comparisons. A version of it is included here for this purpose.

Vital Body Post-Exercise Assessment

Use the following as a guide to assess the post-exercise condition of your vital body.

Exercise: Vital Body Assessment

- Find a quiet place in which you can focus without distraction.

- Be in a seated position, as comfortable as possible.

- Take a couple of slow, deep breaths.

- Gently close your eyes and intentionally shift your attention away from an external focus toward an internal focus, awakening your internal senses.

- Once you have made this shift, again using the power of your intent, consciously focus your attention on your vital body to the best of your ability. Using self-talk, tell yourself that you are now focusing on your vital body.

- Do your best to sense into your vitality, the substance of your vital body, using your capacity to self-sense. How does it feel? What is your vitality level? Energized or depleted? Focus your attention specifically on your vital body and allow yourself to get a palpable experience of it to the best of your ability. There is no right or wrong, just use an attitude of curiosity.

- Then shift to a self-observer mode, where you are looking at your vital body instead of experiencing it. Like a detached detective, examine your vital body, noticing everything you can about it.

- Ask yourself the following questions and jot down your answers on a sheet of paper.

- Spend 30-60 seconds with each of the questions. If nothing comes up as you ask the question, leave it blank and move on to the next.

  - What does your vital body look like?

  - How big is it?

  - What color is it?

  - What shape is it?

  - How does it move?

  - What does it sound like?

- What does it feel like?

- If your vital body could speak, what would it say?

- What is the overall condition of your vital body?

- Take a moment to draw a simple sketch of your vital body.

Compare your current vital body description and sketch with the results you attained from doing this inventory when it first appeared in Chapter 2. If your vital body has improved, congratulations! If not, refer to the guidelines in Chapter 4 to help. Then move on to the emotional body inventory.

Emotional Body Post-Exercise Assessment

Use the following as a guide to assess the post-exercise condition of your emotional body.

Exercise: Emotional Body Assessment

- Find a quiet place in which you can focus without distraction.

- Be in a seated position, as comfortable as possible.

- Take a couple of slow, deep breaths.

- Gently close your eyes and intentionally shift your attention away from an external focus toward an internal focus, awakening your internal senses.

- Once you have made this shift, again using the power of your intent, consciously focus your attention on your emotional body to the best of your ability. Using self-talk, tell yourself that you are now focusing on your emotional body.

- Do your best to sense into your feelings, the substance of your emotional body, using your capacity to self-sense. How does it feel? What is your emotional landscape like? Are you feeling irritated, disappointed, anxious, glad? Focus your attention specifically on your emotional body and allow yourself to get a palpable experience of it to the best of your ability. There is no right or wrong, just use an attitude of curiosity.

- Then shift to a self-observer mode, where you are looking at your emotional body instead of experiencing it. Like a detached detective, examine your emotional body, noticing everything you can about it.

- Ask yourself the following questions and jot down your answers on a sheet of paper.

- Spend 30-60 seconds with each of the questions. If nothing comes up as you ask the question, leave it blank and move on to the next.

- What does your emotional body look like?

  - How big is it?

  - What color is it?

  - What shape is it?

- How does it move?

- What does it sound like?

- What does it feel like?

- If your emotional body could speak, what would it say?

- What is the overall condition of your emotional body?

- Take a moment to draw a sketch of your emotional body.

Compare your current emotional body description and sketch with the results you attained from doing this inventory when it first appeared in Chapter 2. If your emotional body has improved, congratulations! If not, refer to the exercises in Chapter 6 to help. Then move on to the mental body inventory.

Mental Body Post-Exercise Assessment

Use the following as a guide to assess the post-exercise condition of your mental body.

Exercise: Mental Body Assessment

- Find a quiet place in which you can focus without distraction.

- Be in a seated position, as comfortable as possible.

- Slowly, take a couple of deep breaths.

- Gently close your eyes and intentionally shift your attention away from an external focus toward an internal focus, awakening your internal senses.

- Once you have made this shift, again using the power of your intent, consciously focus your attention on your mental body to the best of your ability. Using self-talk, tell yourself that you are now focusing on your mental body.

- Do your best to sense into your thoughts, the substance of your mental body, using your capacity to self-sense. What kind of thoughts are there? What is your mental landscape like? Is it slow, spacious or quiet? Fast, noisy or crowded? Focus your attention specifically on your mental body and allow yourself to get a palpable experience of it to the best of your ability. There is no right or wrong, just use an attitude of curiosity.

- Then shift to a self-observer mode, where you are looking at your mental body instead of experiencing it. Like a detached detective, examine your mental body, noticing everything you can about it.

- Ask yourself the following questions and jot down your answers on a sheet of paper.

- Spend 30-60 seconds with each of the questions. If nothing comes up as you ask the question, leave it blank and move on to the next.

- What does your mental body look like?
  - How big is it?
  - What color is it?
  - What shape is it?
  - How does it move?
  - What does it sound like?
  - What does it feel like?
  - If your mental body could speak, what would it say?
  - What is the overall condition of your mental body?
- Take a moment to draw a sketch of your mental body.

Compare your current mental body description and sketch with the results you attained from doing this inventory when it first appeared in Chapter 2. If your mental body has improved, congratulations! If not, refer to the exercises in Chapter 8 to help. Then move on to the universal body inventory, the final step in the Before and After sequence.

Universal Body Post-Exercise Assessment

Use the following as a guide to assess the post-exercise condition of your universal body.

Exercise: Universal Body Assessment

- Find a quiet place in which you can focus without distraction.

- Be in a seated position, as comfortable as possible.

- Slowly, take a couple of deep breaths.

- Gently close your eyes and intentionally shift your attention away from an external focus toward an internal focus, awakening your internal senses.

- Once you have made this shift, again using the power of your intent, consciously focus your attention on your universal body to the best of your ability. Using self-talk, tell yourself that you are now focusing on your universal body.

- Do your best to sense into the space between your thoughts and feelings, the substance of your universal body, using your capacity to self-sense. How do you experience it? What is your universal landscape like? Can you be in the no-thingness? Focus your attention specifically on your universal body and allow yourself to get a palpable experience of it to the best of your ability. There is no right or wrong, just use an attitude of curiosity.

- Then shift to a self-observer mode, where you are looking at your universal body instead of experiencing it. Like a detached detective, examine your universal body, noticing everything you can about it.

- Ask yourself the following questions and jot down your answers on a sheet of paper.

- Spend 30-60 seconds with each of the questions. If nothing comes up as you ask the question, leave it blank and move on to the next.

- What does your universal body look like?

  - How big is it?

  - What color is it?

  - What shape is it?

  - How does it move?

  - What does it sound like?

  - What does it feel like?

  - If your universal body could speak, what would it say?

  - What is the overall condition of your universal body?

- Take a moment to draw a sketch of your universal body.

Compare your current universal body description and sketch with the results you attained from doing this inventory when it first appeared in Chapter 2. If your universal body has improved, congratulations! If not, refer to the exercises in Chapter 10 to help.

Appendix A

Inergy Body Resources

In keeping with the book's theme, this resource section is organized according to the four bodies. However, as previously mentioned, these delineations are not discreet. There is much overlap, and the inergy system can be entered through any body or several bodies combined. The resources could certainly be categorized differently; some resources could be listed in multiple categories (but are not).

The information below is offered in the spirit of service. Inclusion in the list does not constitute my endorsement. I invite you to take responsibility for your bodies, and educate yourself accordingly, to find what is best for you. The information below was accurate at the time of printing and is subject to change. Thank you for your understanding.

Vital Body Resources

American Association of Acupuncture and Oriental Medicine
PO Box 162340
Sacramento, CA 95816 USA
916-443-4770
www.AAAOMonline.org

www.AntennaSearch.com: Find cell towers and antennas near you

Ayurvedic Institute
11311 Menaul Blvd. NE
Albuquerque, NM 87112 USA
505-291-9698
www.Ayurveda.com

The Body's Burden: Online self-test of household chemical load
http://extras.insidebayarea.com/bodyburden/bodyburden.html

BioInitiative: International consortium of concerned scientists
addressing electromagnetic radiation exposure standards
www.BioInitiative.org
info@bioinitiative.org

Dinshah Health Society
Spectro-Chrome home color therapy
PO Box 707
Malaga NJ 08328 USA
856-692-4686
dinshahhealth@aol.com
www.DinshahHealth.org

Energy Kinesiology Association
5900 CR 90
Red Rock, OK 74651 USA
866-365-4336
www.EnergyK.org
info@EnergyK.org

Healing Touch International, Inc.
445 Union Blvd., Ste. 105
Lakewood, CO 80228 USA
303-989-7982
303-980-8683 - fax
education@HealingTouchInternational.org
www.HealingTouchInternational.org

The International Center for Reiki Training
21421 Hilltop St., Unit #28
Southfield, MI 48033
248-948-8112
248-948-9534 - fax
center@reiki.org
www.Reiki.org

International College of Applied Kinesiology
Applied Kinesiology Center
17A Lenox Pointe NE
Atlanta, GA 30324 USA
404-634-0201
drjohn@akdoc.com
www.ICAK.com

Microwave News
155 East 77th St., Suite 3
New York, NY 10075 USA
212-517-2800
212-734-0316 – fax
www.MicroWaveNews.com
info@microwavenews.com

National Center for Homeopathy
801 North Fairfax St. Ste. 306
Alexandria, VA 22314 USA
703-548-7790
www.Homeopathic.org

Touch For Health Kinesiology Association
3225 West. St. Joseph
Lansing, MI 48917 USA
517-327-9207
admin@TFHKA.org
www.TFHKA.org

World Research Foundation
41 Bell Rock Plaza
Sedona, AZ 86351 USA
928-284-3300
info@wrf.org
www.wrf.org

Emotional Body Resources

Association for Comprehensive Energy Psychology
349 Lancaster Ave., Ste. 101
Haverford, PA 19041 USA
619-861-2237
acep@energypsych.org
www.EnergyPsych.org

The Center for Anger Resolution
2524 Nottingham
Houston, TX 77005 USA
713-526-6650
Newton@AngerBusters.com
www.AngerBusters.com

The Center for Nonviolent Communication
5600 San Francisco Rd. NE Ste. A
Albuquerque, NM 87109 USA
505-244-4140
www.CNVC.org

Consortium for Emotional Intelligence in Organizations
No other contact information available at press time
www.EIConsortium.org

Global Coherence Initiative
Science-based project to advance global heart coherence
www.GLCoherence.org

Daniel Goleman
Author of *Emotional Intelligence* and *Social Intelligence*
No other contact information available at press time
info@danielgoleman.info
www.DanielGoleman.info

Emotional Freedom Technique (EFT)
(Often referred to as "tapping")
PO Box 269
Coulterville, CA 95311 USA
www.EMOFree.com

Emotional Intelligence Information
Research and resources on emotional intelligence
No other contact information available at press time
jack.mayer@unh.edu
www.unh.edu/emotional_intelligence

Institute of HeartMath
Research and education on heart-based living
14700 West Park Ave.
Boulder Creek, CA 95006 USA
831-338-8500
info@heartmath.org
www.HeartMath.org

PAIRS
Practical Application of Intimate Relationship Skills
1056 Creekford Dr.
Weston, FL 33326 USA
954-332-7930
info@pairs.com
www.PAIRS.com

Susan Campbell
Author of *Getting Real*
4373 Hessel Ct.
Sebastopol, CA 95472 USA
707-829-3646
drsusan@susancampbell.com
www.SusanCampbell.com

Tapas Acupressure Technique (TAT)
PO Box 5192
Mooresville, NC 28117 USA
310-378-7381
www.TATLife.net

Mental Body Resources

Dean Radin
Author of *Entangled Minds*
c/o Institute of Noetic Sciences
101 San Antonio Rd.
Petaluma, CA 94952 USA
707-775-3500
dean@noetic.org
www.DeanRadin.com

Inner Clarity (IC)
Transforms limiting belief systems
The work of *Endless Energy* author Debra Greene
c/o MetaComm Media
1215 S. Kihei Rd. Ste. 0-907
Maui, HI 96753 USA
808-874-6441
info@InnerClarity.us
www.InnerClarity.us

Institute of Noetic Sciences
101 San Antonio Rd.
Petaluma, CA 94952 USA
707-775-3500
707-781-7420 – fax
membership@noetic.org
www.noetic.org

International Society for the Study of Subtle Energies
and Energy Medicine (ISSSEEM)
11005 Ralston Rd. , Suite 210
Arvada, CO 80004 USA
303-425-4625
303-425-4685 – fax
wwww.issseem.org
info@issseem.org

Jack Houck
Founder of Psychokinesis Parties
No other contact information available at press time
info@jackhouck.com
www.JackHouck.com

Lynn McTaggart
Author of *The Field* and *Intention Experiment*
Unit 10, Woodman Works
204 Durnsford Rd.
London, England, SW19 8DR
cs@livingthefield.com
www.TheIntentionExperiment.com

Rupert Sheldrake
Developed theories of morphic resonance and morphic fields
No other contact information available at press time
www.Sheldrake.org

Universal Body Resources

Agni Yoga Society
319 West 10th St.
New York, NY 10025 USA
info@agniyoga.org
www.AgniYoga.org

Institute for Global Transformation
Post Office Box 4
4915 Atlanta Hwy.
Flowery Branch, GA 30542
info@IFGT.org
www.IFGT.org

Lucis Trust
120 Wall Street, 24th Floor
New York, NY 10005 USA
212-292-0707
newyork@lucistrust.org
www.LucisTrust.org

The Seven Ray Institute and the
University of the Seven Rays
128 Manhattan Ave.
Jersey Heights, NJ 07307 USA
201-798-7977
sevenray@sevenray.com
www.SevenRay.com

Wisdom Studies
PO Box 130003
Roseville, MN 55113 USA
info@WisdomStudies.com
www.WisdomStudies.com

For a comprehensive listing of resources

Online Wellness Network
San Francisco, CA 94131 USA
415-285-5631
admin@OnlineWellnessNetwork.com
www.OnlineWellnessNetwork.com

Appendix B

Sources for Radiation Detection
and Protection Devices

Gaussmeters and Other EMF Detectors

AlphaLab, Inc.
3005 South 300 West
Salt Lake City, UT 84115 USA
Tel: 801-487-9492
Email: mail@trifield.com
Web: www.TriField.com

Integrity Design and Research Corp.
182 Brown River Rd.
Essex, VT 05452 USA
Tel: 802-872-7116
Email: info@gaussmeter.info
Web: www.GaussMeter.info

Less EMF Inc.
809 Madison Ave.
Albany, NY 12208 USA
Tel: 518-432-1550
Email: lessemf@lessemf.com
Web: www.LessEMF.com

Magnetic Sciences
367 Arlington St.
Acton, MA 01720 USA
Tel: 951-324-7386
Email: info@magneticsciences.com
Web: www.MagneticSciences.com

Personal Energy Devices and Chips

Many people are curious about how such devices could work, so I will attempt a brief explanation here.* Of course, I can't speak for all devices, a full explanation is beyond the scope of this Appendix, and some devices may not work at all. Diode devices tend to work through sympathetic resonance technology, oscillators, and amplifying coils, such as Mobius coils, that emit scaler waves to create sympathetic resonators that enhance your inergy. They work with your vital body to "super-charge" it so it can run more efficiently and have more internal power available to resist harmful influences. Chips tend to contain microchips that produce a stabilizing signal, such as a Schumann resonance frequency, that can give rise to a self-canceling field.

BioPro USA
Corporate Headquarters
1905 Aston Ave.
Ste. 101
Carlsbad, CA 92008 USA
Tel: 760-488-2498
Web: www.BioProTechnology.com
Chips for cell phones and electronics

Q-Link Products
Customer Service
13240 N 20th St.
Ste. 18
Bellevue, WA 98005 USA
Tel: 800-246-2765
Email: support@northwestdir.com
Web: www.Q-LinkProducts.com
Pendants and personal protection devices,
pet protection, room and house protection

Energy Healing Arts
Eyelight Spectrum Products
One Marion Ave. Ste. 311
Mansfield, OH 44903 USA
Tel: 614-297-7001
Web: www.Energy-HealingArts.com
Personal devices, household protection and more

Barrier Methods and Other Cell Phone Protection

Block EMF
2335 Camino Vida Roble, Bldg. B
Carlsbad, CA 92009
Tel: 760-431-8047
Email: customerservice@healthstores.com
Web: www.BlockEMF.com
Barrier devices, personal protection and more

EMF Review
PO Box 670
Lake Forrest, CA 92609 USA
Tel: 888-671-7947
Web: www.EMFReview.com
Hollow tube headsets

RFSafe
Address unavailable at press time
Tel: 727-643-5440
Email: webmaster@rfsafe.com
Web: www.RFSafe.com
Barrier devices, hollow tube headsets, antenna

*For more information, please see James Oschman, *Energy Medicine: The Scientific Basis* (Philadelphia, PA: Churchill Livingston, 2000).

Appendix C

Water Technology

Water Filtration Units

Multipure carries carbon-block countertop, under-the-sink, whole house, and shower filters.

> Multipure Corporation
> 7251 Cathedral Rock Drive
> Las Vegas, NV 89128 USA
> Tel: 702-360-8880, 800-622-9206
> Email: headquarters@MultiPure.com
> Web: www.MultiPure.com

Ionization (structured water) Units*

Water ionization is a complex process involving two things: 1) filtration media that must remove contaminants but not remove the minerals; and 2) electrical parts, including metal components, that must restructure the water without re-contaminating it. The more effective the ionization process, the more stable the water and the longer it can sustain its new structure. Recommended units, such as those below, use platinum-coated titanium electrolytic components. Others on the market using steel or aluminum, both toxic substances, are not recommended.

> Kangen
> Enagic USA Headquarters
> 4115 Spencer St.
> Torrance, CA 90503 USA
> Tel: 310-542-7700
> Web: www.Enagic.com
> Web: www.KangenWtr.com

Jupiter International
ACME Equipment Company
1032 Concert Ave.
Spring Hill FL 34609 USA
Tel: 352-688-3404
Email: Jupiter@acmeequipment.com
Web: www.JupiterIonizers.com

*Thanks to Beverly Rubik, Ph.D., for assistance.

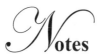

Notes

Chapter 1: Understanding Energy

[1] A.V. Hill, "A Challenge to Biochemists" *Biochim Biophys Acta* 4 (1950): 4-11. Another of Dr. Hill's works on this subject that may be useful: A.V. Hill, *Trails and Trials in Physiology* (London, England: Arnold, 1965).

[2] Beverly Rubik, "The Biofield Hypothesis: Its Biophysical Basis and Role in Medicine" *Journal of Alternative and Complementary Medicine* 8 (2002): 703-717.

[3] Among the sources that describe these energies in various ways are: Dawson Church, *The Genie in Your Genes: Epigenetic Medicine and the New Biology of Intention* (Santa Rosa, CA: Elite, 2007); Richard Gerber, *Vibrational Medicine: New Choices for Healing Ourselves* (Sante Fe, NM: Bear and Company, 1988/1996); Amit Goswami, Richard R. Reed, and Maggie Goswami, *The Self-Aware Universe: How Consciousness Creates the Material World* (New York: Jeremy P. Tarcher/Penguin Putnam, 1993); Charles Krebs, *A Revolutionary Way of Thinking* (Melbourne: Hill of Content, 1998); Bruce Lipton, *The Biology of Belief: Unleashing the Power of Consciousness, Matter, and Miracles* (Santa Rosa, CA: Mountain of Love/Elite, 2005); Lynn McTaggert, *The Field: The Quest for the Secret Force of the Universe* (New York: Harper, 2002); James Oschman, *Energy Medicine: The Scientific Basis* (Philadelphia, PA: Churchill Livingston, 2000); William Tiller, *Science and Human Transformation: Subtle Energies, Intentionality and Consciousness*

(Walnut Creek, CA: Pavior, 1997); William Tiller, Walter Dibble, and J. Gregory Fandel, *Some Science Adventures With Real Magic* (Walnut Creek, CA: Pavior, 2005).

[4] Knight Kiplinger, *The Kiplinger Letter: Forecasts for Management Decisionmaking* [electronic newsletter] (21 December 2008): 85(51), www.kiplingerbiz.com.

[5] L.E. Hebert, P.A. Scherr, J.L. Bienias, D.A. Bennett, and D.A. Evans, "Alzheimer Disease in the U.S. Population: Prevalence Estimates Using the 2000 Census" *Archives of Neurology* 60 (August 2003): 1119–1122.

[6] Patricia M. Barnes, Eve Powell-Griner, Kim McFann and Richard L. Nahin, "Complementary and Alternative Medicine Use Among Adults: United States, 2002" *Seminars in Integrative Medicine* 2 (2004): 54-71.

[7] Rubik, "The Biofield Hypothesis," 708.

[8] The four bodies model is adapted from the work of William Tiller who describes the four dimensions as conjugate/physical (what I refer to as vital/physical), emotional, mental, and spiritual (what I refer to as universal). See, for example, William Tiller, *Psychoenergetic Science: A Second Copernican-Scale Revolution* (Walnut Creek: Pavior, 2007) chapter 7; Tiller, Dibble, and Fandel, *Some Science Adventures With Real Magic*, chapter 3; Tiller, *Science and Human Transformation*, chapter 2. Gerber, *Vibrational Medicine*; and Krebs, *A Revolutionary Way of Thinking*, have expanded on Tiller's work.

[9] See, for example, Rubik, *The Biofield Hypothesis*; Mark Comings, "The Quantum Plenum: Energetics and Sentience" (presentation at the International Society for the Study of Subtle Energies and Energy Medicine conference, Colorado Springs, CO: June 24-30, 2004): www.issseem.org.

[10] Mark Comings, "The Quantum Plenum: Energetics and Sentience" (presentation at the International Society for the Study of Subtle Energies and Energy Medicine conference, Colorado Springs, CO: June 24-30, 2004). This foam contains energy of a magnitude that is 10 to the 104th power. By comparison, the

number of atoms in the visible universe is only about 10 to the 80th power. This foam, when measured in mass, is about 10 to the 94th grams per cubic centimeter. By comparison, just 1 gram of mass includes hundreds of billions of atoms.

[11] See, for example, David Bohm, B.J. Hiley, *The Undivided Universe: An Ontological Interpretation of Quantum Theory* (London: Routledge: 1993); F. David Peat, "Active Information" [retrieved January 27, 2009] www.fdavidpeat.com/ideas/activeinfo. htm; Candice Pert, *Molecules of Emotion: The Science Behind Mind-Body Medicine* (NY: Scribner, 1997); William Tiller, *Psychoenergetic Science* and *Science and Human Transformation*; J.A. Wheeler, "Information, Physics, Quantum: The Search For Links" *Complexity, Entropy, and the Physics of Information, SFI Studies in the Sciences of Complexity*, (Redwood City, CA: Addison-Wesley, 1990); Donald E. Watson, "The Theory of Enformed Gestalts: A Model of Life, Mind, Health" *Advances: The Journal of Mind-Body Health* 13 (1997): 32-36; Donald Watson, "The Enformy Page" [retrieved January 27, 2009] www.enformy. com.

[12] James Oschman, *Energy Medicine in Therapeutics and Human Performance* (Philadelphia, PA: Butterworth Heinemann, 2003); Oschman, *Energy Medicine*; Pert, *Molecules of Emotion*; Tiller, *Psychoenergetic Science*; Watson, "The Enformy Page" www. enformy.com.

[13] Adapted from Amy Choi, "Qi-nesiology Balancing Procedure: Integrating Qigong and Kinesiology" (presentation at the Joint Energy Kinesiology and Touch for Health Conference in Salt Lake City, Utah, June 2007).

[14] Effects such as this have been documented and explained by a number of scientists. See, for example, Valerie Hunt, *Infinite Mind: The Science of Human Vibrations* (Malibu, CA: Malibu Publishing, 1995); Oschman, *Energy Medicine*; Oschman, *Energy Medicine in Therapeutics*; Tiller, *Psychoenergetic Science*; Tiller, Dibble and Fandel, *Some Science Adventures With Real Magic*; Tiller, *Science and Human Transformation*.

Chapter 2: Your Four Bodies

[1] Two major contributors to research on the sense of being stared at are Dean Radin (www.DeanRadin.com) and Rupert Sheldrake (www.Sheldrake.org). You can participate in online experiments at Sheldrake's website. See also, Rupert Sheldrake, "The Sense of Being Stared At Does Not Depend on Known Sensory Cues" *Biology Forum* 93 (2000): 209-224; Dean Radin, "The Sense of Being Stared At: A Preliminary Meta-analysis" *Journal of Consciousness Studies* 12 (2005): 95-100; Dean Radin and Marilyn Schlitz, "Gut Feelings, Intuition, and Emotions: An Exploratory Study" *Journal of Alternative and Complementary Medicine* 11 (2005): 85-91; Dean Radin, "On the Sense of Being Stared At: An Analysis and Pilot Replication" *Journal of the Society for Psychical Research* 68 (2004): 246-253.

[2] Richard Gerber, *Vibrational Medicine: New Choices for Healing Ourselves* (Sante Fe, NM: Bear and Company, 1988/1996); Charles Krebs, *A Revolutionary Way of Thinking* (Melbourne: Hill of Content, 1998); William Tiller, *Psychoenergetic Science: A Second Copernican-Scale Revolution* (Walnut Creek, CA: Pavior, 2007); William Tiller, *Science and Human Transformation: Subtle Energies, Intentionality and Consciousness* (Walnut Creek, CA: Pavior, 1997).

[3] Body cells are information-based and act as amplifiers of experience. For more on this see, for example, Dawson Church, *The Genie in Your Genes: Epigenetic Medicine and the New Biology of Intention* (Santa Rosa, CA: Elite, 2007); Bruce Lipton, *The Biology of Belief: Unleashing the Power of Consciousness, Matter, and Miracles* (Santa Rosa, CA: Mountain of Love/Elite, 2005); James Oschman, *Energy Medicine: The Scientific Basis* (Philadelphia, PA: Churchill Livingston, 2000).

[4] Gerber; *Vibrational Medicine*; Krebs, *A Revolutionary Way of Thinking*; Tiller, *Psychoenergetic Science*; Tiller, *Science and Human Transformation*.

[5] James Oschman builds a strong case for this in *Energy Medicine: The Scientific Basis*. See especially Chapter 13.

[6] See, for example, Dean Radin, "For Whom the Bell Tolls: A Question of Global Consciousness" *Noetic Sciences Review* 63 (2003): 8-13, 44-45; Dean Radin, "Exploratory Study of Relationships Between Physical Entropy and Global Human Attention" *Journal of International Society of Life Information Science* 20 (2002): 690-694; Dean Radin, "Exploring Relationships Between Random Physical Events and Mass Human Attention: Asking For Whom the Bell Tolls" *Journal of Scientific Exploration* 16 (2002): 533-548.

[7] The research substantiating the power of intention has exploded, particularly in terms of its application to health. See, for example, Dean Radin, J. Stone, E. Levine, S. Eskandarnejad, Marilyn Schlitz, L. Kozak, D. Mandel, and G. Hayssen, "Compassionate Intention as a Therapeutic Intervention by Partners of Cancer Patients: Effects of Distant Intention on the Patients' Autonomic Nervous System" *Explore: The Journal of Science and Healing* 4 (2008): 235-243; Dean Radin and Ronald Nelson, "Meta-Analysis of Mind-Matter Interaction Experiments: 1959 – 2000" in *Healing, Intention and Energy Medicine* (London: Harcourt Health Sciences, 2003).

[8] Dean Radin, F. Machado and W. Zangari, "Effects of Distant Healing Intention Through Time and Space: Two Exploratory Studies" *Subtle Energies and Energy Medicine* 11 (2000): 207-240.

[9] William Tiller, "Towards General Experimentation and Discovery in Conditioned Laboratory Spaces: Part I. Experimental pH Change Findings at Some Remote Sites" *The Journal of Alternative and Complementary Medicine* 10 (2004); William Tiller, "Towards General Experimentation and Discovery in Conditioned Laboratory Spaces: Part II, pH Change Experience at Four Remote Sites, 1 Year Later" *The Journal of Alternative and Complementary Medicine* 10 (2004); Dean Radin, R. Taft, and G. Yount, "Possible Effects of Healing Intention on Cell Cultures and Truly Random Events" *Journal of Alternative and Complementary Medicine* 10 (2004): 103-112; William Tiller, Walter Dibble and Michael Kohane, "Towards Objectifying Intention Via Electronic

Devices" *Subtle Energies and Energy Medicine* 8 (1999).
[10] K.A. Martin, S. E. Moritz and C. Hall, "Imagery Use in Sport: A Literature Review and Applied Model" *Sports Psychologist* 13 (1999): 245-68.
[11] Brent Hafen, Keith Karren, Kathryn Frandsen and N. Lee Smith, *Mind Body Health: The Effects of Attitudes, Emotions, and Relationships* (Needham Heights, MA: Allyn and Bacon, 1996), 463-472.
[12] This is a foundational principle of the field of somatics and body-oriented psychotherapies. See, for example, Moshe Feldenkrais, *Awareness Through Movement* (New York, NY: Harper Collins, 1990); Moshe Feldenkrais, *Body Awareness as Healing Therapy* (Berkeley, CA: Frog Ltd. and Somatic Resources, 1997); Thomas Hanna, *Somatics: Reawakening the Mind's Control of Movement, Flexibility, and Health* (Reading, MA: Addison Wesley, 1988).
[13] C. Anderson, D. Keltner, and O. P. John, "Emotional Convergence Between People Over Time" *Journal of Personality and Social Psychology* 84 (May 2003): 1054-1068.
[14] Daniel Goleman, *Emotional Intelligence: Why It Can Matter More Than I.Q.* (New York, NY: Bantam, 1995).

Chapter 3: Your Vital Body

[1] The vital body is not to be confused with the aura. The vital body pervades and powers the physical body, whereas the aura refers to a kind of "halo-effect" produced by the radiatory qualities of your combined vital, emotional, mental and universal bodies. For more on the aura versus the etheric (vital) body, see William Tiller, Walter Dibble, and J. Gregory Fandel, *Some Science Adventures With Real Magic* (Walnut Creek, CA: Pavior, 2005) 222-225. For more on the etheric (vital) body, see, for example, Alice Bailey, *Esoteric Healing* (NY: Lucis, 1971); Richard Gerber, *Vibrational Medicine: New Choices for Healing Ourselves* (Sante Fe, NM: Bear and Company, 1988/1996); Charles Krebs, *A Revolutionary Way of Thinking* (Melbourne: Hill of Content, 1998); Zachary

F. Lansdowne, *The Chakras and Esoteric Healing* (York Beach, Maine: Samuel Weister, 1986); David Tansley, *Radionics and the Subtle Anatomy of Man* (Whitstable, Kent, England: Whitstable Litho: 1972); William Tiller, *Psychoenergetic Science: A Copernican-Scale Revolution* (Walnut Creek, CA: Pavior, 2007); Tiller, *Science and Human Transformation: Subtle Energies, Intentionality and Consciousness* (Walnut Creek, CA: Pavior, 1997); Tiller, Dibble and Fandel, *Some Science Adventures With Real Magic.*

[2] The inergy dimensions of phantom limbs have been documented by various sources. See, for example, Donna Eden, *Energy Medicine* (NY: Jeremy Tarcher/Putnam, 1998) 31-43; David Feinstein, Donna Eden and Gary Craig, *The Promise of Energy Psychology: Revolutionary Tools for Dramatic Personal Change* (NY: Jeremy Tarcher/Putnam, 2005) 197; Gerber, *Vibrational Medicine,* chapter 1.

[3] James Oschman, *Energy Medicine: The Scientific Basis*; James Oschman, *Energy Medicine in Therapeutics and Human Performance*; Tiller, *Psychoenergetic Science*; Tiller, *Science and Human Transformation: Subtle Energies, Intentionality and Consciousness*; Tiller, Dibble and Fandel, *Some Science Adventures With Real Magic.*

[4] Z. H. Cho et al, "New Findings of the Correlation Between Acupoints and Corresponding Brain Cortices Using Functional MRI" *Proceedings of National Academy of Science* 95 (1998): 2670-73. See also Gerber, *Vibrational Medicine,* chapter 4; Oschman, *Energy Medicine in Therapeutics and Human Performance,* chapter 11; Tiller, *Science and Human Transformation,* chapter 3.

[5] Gerber, *Vibrational Medicine,* chapter 10; Valerie Hunt, *Infinite Mind: The Science of Human Vibrations* (Malibu, CA: Malibu Press, 1995); Krebs, *A Revolutionary Way of Thinking,* p. 330-341; Tiller, *Science and Human Transformation,* chapter 3; Tiller, Dibble, and Fandel, *Some Science Adventures With Real Magic,* chapter 6. The centers have also been experientially verified by

various cultures and numerous practitioners. See, for example, Bailey; Barbara Brennan and Jos Smith, *Hands of Light: A Guide to Healing Through the Human Energy Field* (NY: Bantam, 1987); Donna Eden, *Energy Medicine* (NY: Jeremy Tarcher/Putnam, 1998) chapter 5; Carolyn Myss, *Anatomy of the Spirit* (NY: Three Rivers Press, 1996).

[6] CW Leadbeater, *The Chakras* (Wheaton, IL: Quest, 1972).

[7] Bailey; Gerber; Krebs; Lansdowne; Tansley (see endnote 1).

[8] Bailey; Gerber; Krebs; Lansdowne; Tansley; Tiller; Tiller, Dibble, and Fandel (see endnote 1 in this chapter).

[9] Bailey; Gerber; Krebs; Lansdowne; Tansley; Tiller; Tiller, Dibble, and Fandel (see endnote 1 in this chapter)

[10] Gerber, *Vibrational Medicine*; Lansdowne, *The Chakras and Esoteric Healing*; Leadbeater, *The Chakras*.

[11] Gerber, *Vibrational Healing;* Krebs, *A Revolutionary Way of Thinking*; Lansdowne, *The Chakras and Esoteric Healing*; Tansley, *Radionics and the Subtle Anatomy of Man.*

[12] Much has been written on this topic. See, for example, Gerber; Krebs; Lansdowne; Leadbeater; Tansley; Tiller; Tiller, Dibble and Fandel (endnote 1). If you are new to this, Brennan, Eden, and Myss (endnote 5) may be good starting points, although they may differ in their interpretations from the references in endnote 1.

[13] Located on the middle of the forehead, sometimes the brow center is confused with what is called *the third eye.* According to Bailey, a triangular inergy pattern, the third eye, becomes established inside the head through the expansion of consciousness. It involves three centers: the brow and crown along with a minor center near the base of the skull (the alta major center).

[14] Bailey, *Esoteric Healing*; Gerber, *Vibrational Medicine;* Krebs, *A Revolutionary Way of Thinking*; Lansdowne, *The Chakras and Esoteric Healing.*

[15] Dawson Church, *The Genie in Your Genes: Epigenetic Medicine and the New Biology of Intention* (Santa Rosa, CA: Elite, 2007); Bruce Lipton, *The Biology of Belief: Unleashing the Power of*

Consciousness, Matter, and Miracles (Santa Rosa, CA: Mountain of Love/Elite, 2005).

[16] Gerber, *Vibrational Medicine;* Krebs, *A Revolutionary Way of Thinking.*

[17] William Tiller, *Psychoenergetic Science*, chapter 7; Tiller, Dibble and Fandel, *Some Science Adventures With Real Magic*, chapter 3.

[18] If you are more visually oriented, artist Alex Grey has done an amazing job of painting the physical/etheric interface: www.AlexGrey.com.

Chapter 4: Steps to a Healthy Vital Body

[1] James Oschman, "Energy Medicine: Why You Can Do What You Do" (presentation at the Energy Kinesiology Conference, Salt Lake City, UT: June 6-9, 2007). Jim was quoting Swedish physician and EMF researcher Olle Johansson, a professor at Stockholm's Karolinska Institute who has been researching EMFs for 30 years. A 15 part interview with Johansson on the effects of Mobile Phone Radiation (2008) is available on YouTube: http://ru.youtube.com/view_play_list?p=434FAFD70A66A05F. See also www.MicroWaveNews.com.

[2] Sean Michael Kerner, "Cell Phones Rising" July, 2005, *InternetNews: Realtime IT News* [retrieved 27 Oct. 2008]: www.internetnews.com/wireless/article.php/3522076.

[3] *Facebook Statistics* [retrieved 2 Jan. 2009]: www.FaceBook.com. As an interactive medium, cyberspace changes quickly. By the time this book goes to press most likely a new social networking giant will have emerged.

[4] James Oschman, *Energy Medicine: The Scientific Basis* (Philadelphia, PA: Churchill Livingston, 2000).

[5] Geoffrey Lean, "Warning: Using a Mobile Phone While Pregnant Can Seriously Damage Your Baby" *The Independent*, May 18, 2008.

[6] BioInitiative, "BioInitiative Report: A Rationale for a Biologically-Based Public Exposure Standard for Electromagnetic

Fields (ELF and RF)" August 31, 2007, *BioInitiative Report* [retrieved 5 Sept. 2007]: www.BioInitiative.org; Another clearinghouse for valuable information about EMF/RFR is www. MicrowaveNews.com.

[7] Oschman, *Energy Medicine,* 201-203, 212, 251.

[8] Oschman, *Energy Medicine*, 201.

[9] EMF Review, "Pittsburgh Cancer Institute's Cell Phone Advisory: 10 Great Tips" *EMF Review* [retrieved 3 Jan. 2009]: www. EMFReview.com/protect-your-family/index.html.

[10] Independent research shows improvement in blood cell integrity, tissue cell resilience, skin conductivity, muscle strength, stabilizing electrical activities of the brain, and lowered anxiety with the Q-Link brand SRT "sympathetic resonance technology" [retrieved 1 Feb. 2009]: www.Q-LinkProducts.com/h_science_research. shtml.

[11] David Pozar, *Microwave Engineering* (Cambridge, MA: Addison-Wesley, 1993). Electromagnetic spectrum delineations are fairly arbitrary and used differently in various fields. I have used Pozar's broader definition for ease of writing while the Institute of Electrical and Electronics Engineers (IEEE) definition starts at 1000 MHz, still inclusive of wireless internet, GPS systems, satellite phones, Bluetooth, and some cell phones. 1000 MHz is 1000 megahertz and 1000 MHz equals 1 GHz or gigahertz.

[12] Oschman. *Energy Medicine,* 210.

[13] General Data Resources, Inc. [retrieved 31 Dec. 2008]: www. AntennaSearch.com. This number reflects cell towers and antennas 200 feet or higher, for the most part. To find cell tower and antenna locations nearby your home or workplace, go to www. AntennaSearch.com. At the time of printing, this service was free.

[14] Create Healthy Homes: Environmental Design and Inspection Services, "Research Citations on the Health Hazards of Cell Phones, Cordless Telephones and Wireless Internet (WiFi)" [retrieved 7 Jan. 2009]: www.CreateHealthyHomes.com/cellphone _risks.php; Radio Frequency Safe, "DNA and the Microwave Effect" *Radio Frequency Safe* [retrieved 7 Jan. 2009]: www.rfsafe.

com/research/rf_hazards/dna_ damage/microwave_effect.html.
15 Create Healthy Homes; Radio Frequency Safe.
16 Adapted from EMF Review, "Pittsburgh Cancer Institute's Cell Phone Advisory."
17 Adapted from Create Healthy Homes: Environmental Design and Inspection Service; Radio Frequency Safe.
18 Julius Goepp, "The Link Between Autism and Low Levels of Vitamin D" *Life Extension* 15 (April, 2009) 79-87; Iain Lang et al, "Vitamin D and Cognitive Impairment" *Journal of Geriatric Psychology and Neurology* (Jan., 2009).
19 Darius Dinshah, *Lighting* 95 (Dinshah Health Society Newsletter, June 29, 2007) and *Illumination* 98 (April 18, 2008). www.DinshahHealth.org.
20 Dinshah, 95, 97-98.
21 Dinshah, 95.
22 Darius Dinshah, *Let There Be Light: Practical Manual for Spectro-Chrome Therapy* (Malaga: NJ, 2003). Dinshah was one of the foremost researchers and practitioners of color-light therapy. His results are profound and compelling. www.DinshahHealth.org.
23 Michael Pollan, *In Defense of Food: An Eater's Manifesto* (New York, NY: Penguin, 2008).
24 Mike Adams, "Hidden Dangerous Ingredients in Your Groceries" *NewsTarget Insider* [electronic newsletter] (16 Oct. 2007): www.NewsTarget.com.
25 Institute for Responsible Technology, "Genetically Modified Ingredients Overview" [retrieved 5 Jan. 2009] www.ResponsibleTechnology.org/GMFree/AboutGMFoods.index.cfm.
26 Bruce Lipton, *The Biology of Belief* (Santa Rosa, CA: Mountain of Love/Elite, 2005); Oschman, *Energy Medicine*, (Philadelphia, PA: Churchill Livingston, 2000) p. 221-223; Understanding cells as information sensors also helps explain how kinesiology muscle testing works.
27 Dawson Church, *The Genie in Your Genes: Epigenetic Medicine and the New Biology of Intention* (Santa Rosa, CA: Elite, 2007); Lipton, *The Biology of Belief*; Oschman, *Energy Medicine*,

especially chapter 3; Oschman, *Energy Medicine in Therapeutics and Human Performance.*

[28] For a free online self-test of your body's chemical burden go to: http://extras.insidebayarea.com/bodyburden/bodyburden.html. See also Nena Baker, *The Body Toxic: How the Hazardous Chemistry of Everyday things Threatens Our Health*, NY: North Point, 2008).

[29] Institute for Responsible Technology.

[30] James Oschman, "Energy Medicine: Why You Can Do What You Do" (presentation at the Joint Energy Kinesiology and Touch for Health Conference, Salt Lake City, UT: June, 2007).

[31] Star Trek, The Next Generation, "Home Soil" Episode 17.

[32] Karl Maret, "Fields, Physics and Subtle Energies" (presentation at the International Society for the Study of Subtle Energies and Energy Medicine conference, Colorado Springs, CO: June, 2004).

[33] Oschman, *Energy Medicine,* 199.

[34] Richard Gerber, *Vibrational Medicine: New Choices for Healing Ourselves* (Sante Fe, NM: Bear and Company, 1988/1996).

[35] Masaru Emoto, *Messages In Water* (Hillsboro, OR: Beyond Words, 2004); Dean Radin, G. Hayssen, Masaru Emoto, and T. Kizu, "Double-blind Test of the Effects of Distant Intention on Water Crystal Formation" *Explore: The Journal of Science and Healing* 2(5) (2006): 408-411.

[36] Paul Pitchford, *Healing With Whole Foods* (Berkeley: North Atlantic Books, 1993).

[37] Rob Stein, "Scientists Find Out What Losing Sleep Does to a Body" *Washington Post* (Oct, 9, 2005) A1.

[38] Research Matters, "Lack of Sleep Disrupts Brain's Emotional Controls" National Institutes of Health (Nov. 5, 2007).

[39] Alice Bailey, *Esoteric Healing* (New York, NY: Lucis, 1971).

[40] Dr. Janel Guyette, M.D., personal conversation.

[41] Gerald Fletcher, A. Nasha, and Dimitrios Trichopoulos, "Midday Nap Cuts Heart Deaths" *Archives of Internal Medicine* 167 (Feb. 12, 2007): 296-301.

[42] Adapted from Grethe Fremming and Rolf Havsboel, "Clearing: Centering" in *Transformational Kinesiology: Foundation* (Kirke,

Hyllinge, Denmark, 1993).

[43] Adapted from Paul and Gail Dennison, *Brain Gym: Simple Activities for Whole Brain Learning* (Ventura, CA: Edu-Kinesthetics, 1986).

[44] It connects Central meridian (CV) with Governing meridian.

[45] Adapted from John Thie and Matthew Thie, "The Balancing Process: Switch On" in *Touch for Health: A Practical Guide to Natural Health With Acupressure Touch* (Camarillo, CA: DeVorss, 2005), used with permission. The entire Touch For Health program is recommended for vital body health. www.Touch4Health.com.

[46] The collar indentations are called K-27s because they correspond to point 27 on the kidney meridian.

[47] The point above the lip corresponds to the endpoint of Central meridian (often called Conception Vessel in Chinese Medicine) and the point below the lip corresponds to the endpoint of Governing meridian.

[48] This area corresponds to the starting point of Governing meridian.

Chapter 5: Your Emotional Body

[1] Vincent Felitti, Robert Anda, Dale Nordenberg, David Williamson, Alison Sptiz, Valerie Edwards, Mary Koss, and James Marks, "Relationship of Childhood Abuse and Household Dysfunction to Many of the Leading Causes of Death in Adults: The Adverse Childhood Experiences (ACE) Study," *American Journal of Preventative Medicine* 14(4) (May, 1998).

[2] Adapted from David Hawkins, "Map of Consciousness" *Power Versus Force: The Hidden Determinants of Human Behavior* (Sedona, AZ: Veritas, 1995) 52-53. Hawkins derived the calibration figures from kinesiological muscle testing research spanning 20 years.

[3] Dawson Church, *The Genie in Your Genes: Epigenetic Medicine and the New Biology of Intention* (Santa Rosa, CA: Elite, 2007); Bruce Lipton, *The Biology of Belief* (Santa Rosa, CA: Elite, 2005);

Candice Pert, *Molecules of Emotion* (NY: Touchstone, 1997).

[4] As outlined previously, our body cells are an excitable medium, much like liquid crystals, that act as amplifiers of experience. Perception plays a large role in "programming" our cells. For more on this see, for example, Church; Lipton; Pert.

[5] Richard Gerber, *Vibrational Medicine: New Choices for Healing Ourselves* (Sante Fe, NM: Bear and Company, 1988/1996) 151-152.

[6] Daniel Wegner, D.J. Schneide, S. Carter and T. White, "Paradoxical Effects of Thought Suppression" *Journal of Personality and Social Psychology* 53 (1987): 5-13.

[7] J. Abramowitz, D. Tolin, G. P. Street, "Paradoxical Effects of Thought Suppression: A Meta-Analysis of Controlled Studies" *Clinical Psychology Review* 21 (2001): 683-703.

[8] Brent Hafen, Keith Karren, Kathryn Frandsen, and N. Lee Smith, *Mind Body Health: The Effects of Attitudes, Emotions, and Relationships* (Needham Heights, MA: Allyn and Bacon, 1996) 111-112, 154-56, 174-179.

[9] Hafen, Karren, Frandsen, and Smith, 160-164.

[10] Carolyn Myss, *Why People Don't Heal and How They Can* (New York, NY: Three Rivers Press, 1997).

[11] Newton Hightower, *Anger Busting 101* (Houston, TX: Bayou Publishing, 2002).

[12] The Institute of HeartMath has been researching heart-brain interactions and heart coherence for over 15 years with extraordinary findings about the efficacy of love: www.HeartMath. org. See also Church, *The Genie in Your Genes*; Lipton, *The Biology of Belief*; Glen Rein, Mike Atkinson and Rollin McCraty, "The Physiological and Psychological Effects of Compassion and Anger" *Journal of Advancement in Medicine* 8(2) (1995): 87-105.

Chapter 6: Steps to a Healthy Emotional Body

[1] R.C. Kessler, W.T. Chiu, O. Demler, and E.E. Walters, "Prevalence, Severity, and Comorbidity of Twelve-Month DSM-

IV Disorders in the National Comorbidity Survey Replication (NCS-R) *Archives of General Psychiatry* 62(6) (June, 2005): 617-27.

[2] Carlos Blanco, Mayumi Okuda, Crystal Wright, Deborah S. Hasin, Bridget F. Grant, Shang-Min Liu, and Mark Olfson, "Mental Health of College Students and Their Non–College-Attending Peers: Results From the National Epidemiologic Study on Alcohol and Related Conditions" *Archives of General Psychiatry* 65(12) (2008): 1429-1437. Over 5000 young adults aged 19-25 were interviewed for this study in 2001-02.

[3] Encarnacion Pyle, "Drugged Into Submission: Even Babies Are Treated As Mentally Ill" *The Columbus Dispatch* (Columbus, Ohio, April 25, 2005). The state of Ohio paid out over $65 million in 2004 for 40,000 kids to take medications for anxiety, depression, hyperactivity and aggressive behavior. This included 696 babies—newborns to 3 years old—who received sedatives and mood-altering drugs through Medicaid. Many of these drugs have not been tested on children. FDA warnings list side effects ranging from headaches and nausea to heart attacks, liver damage, suicidal ideations, and sudden death, as in the case of an 11 year old who died of a heart attack, the day after she took her increased Ritalin dosage which had been doubled by her doctor.

[4] Daniel Goleman, *Emotional Intelligence: Why It Can Matter More Than IQ* (NY: Bantam, 1995).

[5] Stuart Wolpert, "Putting Feelings Into Words Produces Therapeutic Effects in the Brain" *UCLA Newsroom* (June 21, 2007) [retrieved January 10, 2009]: www.newsroom.ucla.edu/portal/ucla/Putting-Feelings-Into-Words-Produces-8047.aspx.

[6] Adapted from Lori Gordon, "Emptying the Jug" in *PAIRS Passage to Intimacy: A Weekend Workshop* (The PAIRS Foundation, Westen, FL: 2001): www.pairs.com.

[7] The version included here differs from the original EFT and is not meant to represent the original technique.

[8] Dawson Church, "The Genie in Your Genes" (presentation at the Joint Energy Kinesiology and Touch for Health Conference,

Sacramento, CA. June 2008): www.SoulMedicineInstitute.org. The primary site for this study is Marshall University Medical School and results are due out in 2010.

[9] Gary Craig, Founder of EFT, is extremely generous with EFT. You can go to his www.EmoFree.com website and download free manuals and instructions.

[10] A more detailed discussion of how the tapping process works is found in David Feinstein, Donna Eden, and Gary Craig, *The Promise of Energy Psychology: Revolutionary Tools for Dramatic Personal Change* (NY: Jeremy Tarcher/Penguin, 2005).

[11] Eye movements are effectively used in a variety of therapies. Most of the work on eye movement and brain functioning comes from Neuro-Linguistic Programming (www.PureNLP.com). Eye rotations are used in Eye Movement Desensitization and Reprocessing therapy (www.EMDR.com) and in various kinesiologies (www.EnergyK.org).

[12] Goleman, *Emotional Intelligence*, 115.

[13] Adapted from Torkum Saraydarian, *The Psyche and Psychism* (Sedona, AZ: Aquarian Educational Group, 1981).

[14] Paul Maclean, *The Triune Brain in Evolution: Role in Paleocerebral Functions* (NY: Plenum Press, 1990); Saraydarian, *The Psyche and Psychism*.

[15] Digital Pharmaceutics: www.MedicalMusicGroup.com. Also the Monroe Institute has research on their Hemispheric Synchronization music: www.MonroeInstitute.com.

[16] The Institute of HeartMath has developed a portable feedback device that is shown to train you in attaining and sustaining high frequency (heart-coherent) emotional states: www.HeartMath.org.

Chapter 7: Your Mental Body

[1] Jack Houck's website is a good resource for information on remote viewing, psychokinesis (PK), PK parties, and other psi phenomena: www.JackHouck.com.

[2] Hal Puthoff, "CIA-Initiated Remote Viewing at Stanford

Research Institute," [retrieved 19 Jan. 2009] www.
BioMindSuperPowers.com/Pages/CIA-InitiatedRV.html. These
documents were declassified in July 1995.
[3] The study of intention has exploded with supportive research.
See, for example, Lynn McTaggart, *The Intention Experiment:
Using Your Thoughts to Change Your Life and the World*
(New York, NY: Free Press, 2007); Ronald Nelson and Dean
Radin, "Statistically Robust Anomalous Effects: Replication in
Random Event Generator Experiments" in *Basic Research in
Parapsychology* (Jefferson, NC: McFarland & Company, 2001);
Dean Radin, *Entangled Minds: Extrasensory Experiences in a
Quantum Reality* (New York, NY: Paraview, 2006); Dean Radin,
G. Hayssen, and J. Walsh, "Effects of Intentionally Enhanced
Chocolate on Mood," *Explore: The Journal of Science and Healing*
3 (2007): 485-492; Dean Radin, G. Hayssen, Masaru Emoto and
T. Kizu, "Double-Blind Test of the Effects of Distant Intention
on Water Crystal Formation" *Explore: The Journal of Science
and Healing* 2 (2006): 408-411; William Tiller, *Psychoenergetic
Science: A Second Copernican-Scale Revolution* (Walnut Creek,
CA: Pavior, 2007); William Tiller, Walter Dibble, J, Gregory
Fandel, *Some Science Adventures With Real Magic* (Walnut
Creek, CA: Pavior, 2005); William Tiller, *Science and Human
Transformation: Subtle Energies, Intentionality and Consciousness*
(Walnut Creek, CA: Pavior, 1997).
[4] William Tiller, Michael Kohane, Michael Dibble and Walter
Dibble, "Can an Aspect of Consciousness be Imprinted into an
Electronic Device?" *Integrative Physiological and Behavioral
Science* (April 1, 2000); Tiller, *Psychoenergetic Science*, chapter
3; Tiller, Dibble and Fandel, *Some Science Adventures With Real
Magic*, chapter 2.
[5] Tiller, Kohane, Dibble and Dibble, 30-31.
[6] Jack Houck summarizes 22 years of research in "Material
Deformation By Intention," [retrieved 25 Jan. 2009] www.
JackHouck.com/articles.shtml; McTaggart; Radin, *Entangled
Minds*; Dean Radin, *The Conscious Universe: The Scientific*

Truth of Psychic Phenomena (San Francisco, CA: HarperCollins, 1997); Rupert Sheldrake, *The Sense of Being Stared At and Other Unexplained Powers of the Human Mind* (New York, NY: Three Rivers, 2003); Sheldrake, *The Presence of the Past: Morphic Resonance and the Habits of Nature* (South Paris, Maine: Park Street Press, 1995).

[7] The Institute of Biosensory Psychology is in St. Petersburg, Russia: www.BioSens.ru.

[8] Annie Besant and C.W. Leadbeater, *Thought-Forms* (Wheaton, Ill: Quest, 1986).

[9] Besant and Leadbeater's book has full color pictorials of various thought-forms.

[10] Houck, "Remote Viewing."

[11] Tiller, *Psychoenergetic Science.*

[12] The link between emotional intensity, high neuroticism, and dementia is well established. See, for example, Hui-Xin Wang, A. Karp, A. Herlitz, M. Crowe, I. Kåreholt, B. Winblad, and L. Fratiglioni, "Personality and Lifestyle in Relation to Dementia Incidence" *Journal of Neurology* 72 (Jan. 13, 2009): 253-259.

Chapter 8: Steps to a Healthy Mental Body

[1] The psychology of the seven types has been advanced by multiple sources. See, for example, Michael Robbins, *Tapestry of the Gods: The Seven Rays, An Esoteric Key to Understanding Human Nature* (Jersey Heights, NJ: University of the Seven Rays, 1988).

[2] Masaru Emoto, *The Hidden Messages In Water* (Hillsboro, OR: Beyond Words, 2004).

[3] Adapted from Grethe Fremming and Rolf Havsboel, "Chakra Balance," in *Transformational Kinesiology: 1* (Kirke, Hyllinge, Denmark, 1993).

[4] This exercise is called the *Pillow Method* and was devised by a group of Japanese students for conflict resolution. The name refers to the rectangular shape of a pillow, with four sides and one center position on which to rest your head. The exercise consists of five

steps that could be seen to correspond to the five pillow positions.
⁵ Adapted from Grethe Fremming and Rolf Havsboel, "Habit
Change," in *Transformational Kinesiology: 3* (Kirke, Hyllinge,
Denmark, 1993).
⁶ Inspired by Rupert Sheldrake's online experiments: www.
Sheldrake.org.
⁷ If you want to participate in similar experiments online, check out
www.Sheldrake.org, the website of Rupert Sheldrake, the biologist
who devised the theory of morphic fields and morphic resonance
which describes a living, developing, interconnected universe.

Chapter 9: Your Universal Body
¹ This was the joint Energy Kinesiology and Touch for Health
conference: www.EnergyK.org.
² See, for example, B. Braun, "Psychophysiologic Phenomena in
Multiple Personality and Hypnosis" *American Journal of Clinical
Hypnosis* 26 (1983): 124-135; P. Coons, et al., "EEG Studies of
Two Multiple Personalities and a Control" *Archives of General
Psychiatry* 39 (July, 1982): 823; Daniel Goleman, "Probing the
Enigma of Multiple Personality" *N.Y.Times* (June 28, 1988):
C1, C13; F. Putnam, "The Psychophysiological Investigation
of Multiple Personality Disorder" *Psychiatric Clinics of North
America* 7 (1984): 31-39.
³ Dawson Church, *The Genie in Your Genes: Epigenetic Medicine
and the New Biology of Intention* (Santa Rosa, CA: Elite, 2007);
Bruce Lipton, *The Biology of Belief: Unleashing the Power of
Consciousness, Matter, and Miracles* (Santa Rosa, CA: Mountain
of Love/Elite, 2005).
⁴ Adapted from David Hawkins, "Map of Consciousness" *Power
Versus Force: The Hidden Determinants of Human Behavior*
(Sedona, AZ: Veritas, 2004) 52-52. Hawkins derived the
calibration figures from kinesiological muscle testing research
spanning 20 years.
⁵ Carol Davis, "Consciousness Field Pupillary Response"

[retrieved January 24, 2009] http://cf-pr.com.

[6] Rollin McCraty, M. Atkinson, and R. Bradley, "Electrophysiological Evidence of Intuition: The Surprising Role of the Heart" (presentation at the International Society for the Study of Subtle Energies and Energy Medicine conference, June 24-30, 2004). See also Institute of HeartMath research: www. HeartMath.org/research/overview.html.

[7] See, for example, Dean Radin, *Entangled Minds: Extrasensory Experiences in a Quantum Reality* (New York, NY: Paraview, 2006); Dean Radin, *The Conscious Universe: The Scientific Truth of Psychic Phenomena* (San Francisco, CA: HarperCollins, 1997); Rupert Sheldrake, *The Sense of Being Stared At and Other Unexplained Powers of the Human Mind* (New York, NY: Three Rivers, 2003); Sheldrake, *The Presence of the Past: Morphic Resonance and the Habits of Nature* (South Paris, Maine: Park Street Press, 1995).

[8] Lyall Watson, *Lifetide* (New York, NY: Bantam, 1980); Ken Keyes, *The Hundredth Monkey* (Mill Valley, CA: Vision Books International, 1981).

[9] This is an example of what Biologist Rupert Sheldrake calls *morphic resonance* that is the result of over-arching morphic fields that unite us: www.Sheldrake.org.

[10] The Global Union of Scientists for Peace (GUSP), is dedicated to researching and advancing technologies of consciousness that have been scientifically shown to neutralize acute social tensions. Their methods are the most thoroughly tested and rigorously verified technologies of defense on the planet: www.GUSP.org.

[11] J. Davies and C. Alexander, "Alleviating Political Violence Through Reducing Collective Tension: Impact Assessment Analyses of the Lebanon War" *Journal of Social Behavior and Personality* 17(1) (2005): 285–338; J. Davies, C. Alexander, and D. Orme-Johnson, "Alleviating Political Violence Through Enhancing Coherence in Collective Consciousness: Impact Assessment Analyses of the Lebanon War" *Journal of the Iowa Academy of Science* 95(1) (1988): 1.

[12] John Hagelin, D. Orme-Johnson, M. Rainforth, K. Cavanaugh, and C. Alexander, "Results of the National Demonstration Project to Reduce Violent Crime and Improve Governmental Effectiveness in Washington, D.C." *Social Indicators Research* 47 (1999): 153-201. See also M. Dillbeck, G. Landrith, and D. Orme-Johnson, "The Transcendental Meditation Program and Crime Rate Change in a Sample of Forty-Eight Cities" *Journal of Crime and Justice* 4 (1981): 25–45.

[13] Menas Kafatos and Thalia Kafatou, *Looking In, Seeing Out: Consciousness and Cosmos* (Wheaton, IL: Quest Books, 1991) 60, 64-65, 102.

Chapter 10: Steps to a Healthy Universal Body

[1] Adapted from Ken Wilber's ingenious identification and articulation of the pre/trans fallacy in *Sex, Ecology, Spirituality* (Boston, MA: Shambhala, 1995).

[2] Adapted from Charles and Barbara Whitfield's insightful identification of spiritual bypassing, later advanced by James Welwood. See, for example, Charles Whitfield, *Healing the Child Within* (Deerfield Beach, FL: Health Communications, 1987); Whitfield, *Co-dependence: Healing the Human Condition* (Deerfield Beach, FL, Health Communications, 1991); Barbara Whitfield, *Spiritual Awakenings* (Deerfield Beach, FL, Health Communications, 1995); James Welwood, *Toward a Psychology of Awakening* (Boston, MA: Shambhala, 2000).

[3] Adapted from Grethe Fremming and Rolf Havsboel, "Alignment," in *Transformational Kinesiology: 1* (Kirke, Hyllinge, 1993). Inspired by Torkum Saraydarian, *The Psyche and Psychism,* p. 865, and Roberto Assagioli's psychosynthesis.

[4] Adapted from Fremming and Havsboel, "The Chakras."

[5] Adapted from David Hawkins, "Map of Consciousness" *Power Versus Force: The Hidden Determinants of Human Behavior* (Sedona, AZ: Veritas, 2004) 52-52. Hawkins derived the calibration figures from kinesiological muscle testing research

spanning 20 years.

[6] Adapted from Torkum Saraydarian, *The Psyche and Psychism* (Aquarian Educational Group, Sedona, AZ: 1981) 827.

[7] Adapted from Fremming and Havsboel, "Eternity," in *Transformational Kinesiology: 5* (Kirke, Hyllinge, Denmark, 1994).

[8] Inner Clarity (IC) is a consciousness-based inergy modality developed by the author: www.InnerClarity.us.

[9] Adapted from Torkum Saraydarian, *The Science of Becoming Oneself*, (Aquarian Educational Group, Sedona, AZ: 1996).

About the Author

Debra has long been interested in how the bodymind system communicates within itself and how we interact with it. Her background is in communication and somatics (bodymind integration), having earned her Ph.D. from Ohio State University. She is the founder of Inner Clarity (IC), a modality that uses energy-based techniques to enact significant progress quickly and efficiently.

IC is a consciousness-based approach in which energy kinesiology (muscle testing) is used to access information from the bodymind system. Questions are asked and answers derived in a way that disassembles defenses and easily reveals the core of the issue. An integrative approach, IC employs holistic counseling and a variety of energy balancing techniques to transform limitations in the vital/physical, emotional, mental and universal bodies. IC combines the art of energy testing with the science of subtle energies for *"the most amount of change in the least amount of time."*

Debra is known for her ability to get to the core of energy imbalances and facilitate lasting improvement. An engaging and accessible speaker, she enjoys sharing her knowledge with others. She teaches and has a private practice on Maui, where she lives, and in the San Francisco Bay area, her second home. Please visit her on the web.

www.DebraGreene.com

- Practice groups
- Free downloads
- Speaking events
- Online community
- Free newsletter
- Workshops and trainings
- Sessions with Debra